THE CARTOON GUIDE TO
SEX

THE CARTOON GUIDE TO

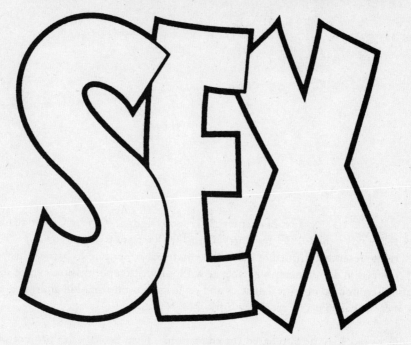

SEX

Larry Gonick and Christine DeVault

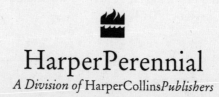

HarperPerennial
A Division of HarperCollinsPublishers

HarperCollins books may be purchased for educational, business, or sales promotional use. For information please write: Special Markets Department, HarperCollins Publishers, Inc., 10 E. 53rd Street, New York, NY 10022

FIRST EDITION

Designed by Larry Gonick

Library of Congress Cataloging-in-Publication Data
Gonick, Larry.
    The cartoon guide to sex / Larry Gonick and Christine DeVault.
       p.   cm.
    Includes bibliographical references.
    ISBN 0–06–273431–8
    1. Sex—Caricatures and cartoons. 2. American wit and humor,
Pictorial. I. DeVault, Christine. II. Title.
  NC1763.S5G66   1999
    306.7'02'07—dc21   99-24253

99 00 01 02 03 RRD 10 9 8 7 6 5 4 3 2 1

WARNING!!

DEAR READER,

CREATING A CARTOON GUIDE TO SEX RAISED A CERTAIN ARTISTIC PROBLEM FOR THE AUTHORS. IN A GRAPHIC MEDIUM, WE WONDERED, EXACTLY HOW GRAPHIC SHOULD WE MAKE IT? SHOULD WE USE SENSITIVE LINE DRAWINGS? BAWDY CARTOONS? FIG LEAVES?

THE QUESTION BARELY AROSE IN SOME CHAPTERS, ESPECIALLY THE ONES DEALING WITH THE SEXUAL ISSUES THAT TEND TO COME UP WHILE WE'RE FULLY CLOTHED: THINGS LIKE COMMUNICATION, LOVE, CHILDHOOD DEVELOPMENT, AND EVEN ILLNESS AND CRIME.

BUT LET'S FACE IT: IT'S A BOOK ABOUT SEX! ONE OF OUR MAIN POINTS IS THAT OPENNESS AND FRANKNESS ABOUT HUMAN SEXUALITY ARE GOOD THINGS. NOT LOOKING AT IT WON'T MAKE IT GO AWAY. HOW THEN COULD WE POSSIBLY NOT ADDRESS THE SUBJECT, AS IT WERE, HEAD ON?

THIS BOOK CONTAINS EXPLICIT MATERIAL.

THERE ARE SENSITIVE LINE DRAWINGS, LOTS OF CARTOONS, AND NO FIG LEAVES; FOR EXAMPLE, ON PAGES 14, 21, 24, 40, 46, 47, 112, 138, 139, 140, 141, 143, 144, 146, 157......
SOME OF YOU MAY WANT TO CLOSE YOUR EYES WHEN YOU COME TO THESE PAGES. THE REST OF YOU CAN GO THERE RIGHT NOW. OH, YOU ALREADY DID?

FINALLY, IN CASE YOU'RE EASILY EMBARRASSED, YOU CAN MAKE YOUR OWN DUST JACKET BY CUTTING OUT A RECTANGLE FROM A BROWN PAPER BAG AND FOLDING IT ALONG THE DOTTED LINES AS SHOWN. NOW YOU CAN READ THE BOOK ON THE BUS, AT THE BEACH, OR AT THE CHURCH SOCIAL.

ENJOY!!

— THE AUTHORS

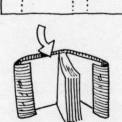

CONTENTS

· CHAPTER 1 ·

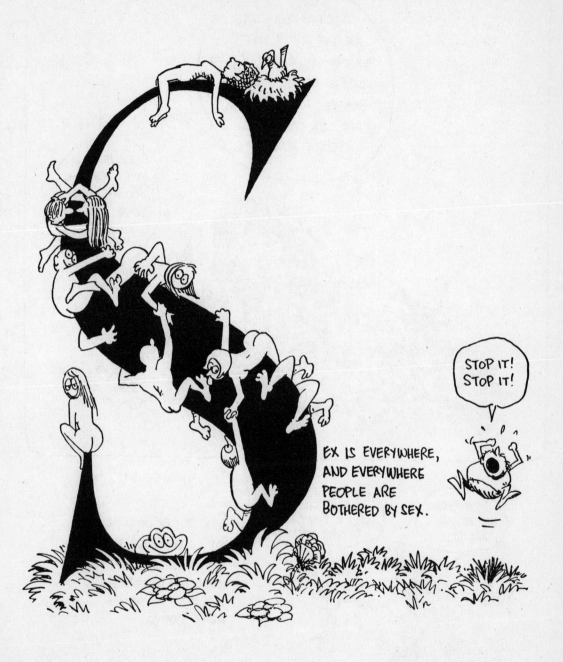

EX IS EVERYWHERE, AND EVERYWHERE PEOPLE ARE BOTHERED BY SEX.

STOP IT! STOP IT!

SEX IS FULL OF PARADOXES
LIKE THAT.

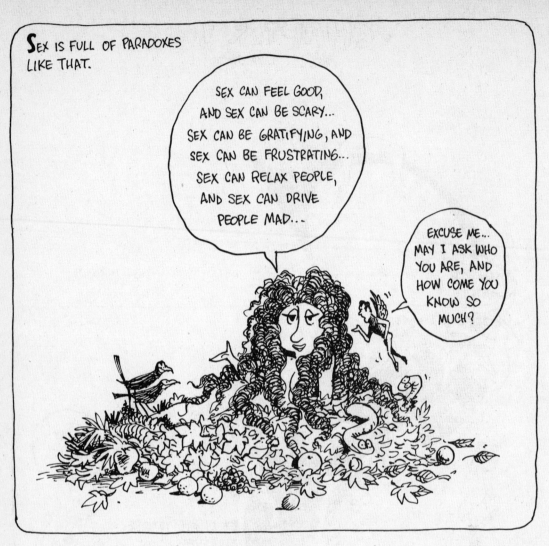

SEX CAN FEEL GOOD,
AND SEX CAN BE SCARY...
SEX CAN BE GRATIFYING, AND
SEX CAN BE FRUSTRATING...
SEX CAN RELAX PEOPLE,
AND SEX CAN DRIVE
PEOPLE MAD...

EXCUSE ME...
MAY I ASK WHO
YOU ARE, AND
HOW COME YOU
KNOW SO
MUCH?

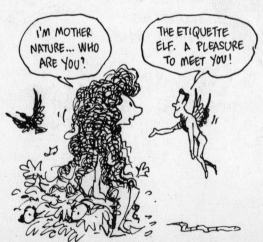

I'M MOTHER
NATURE... WHO
ARE YOU?

THE ETIQUETTE
ELF. A PLEASURE
TO MEET YOU!

SEX CAN BE GOOD OR
BAD, INTENSE OR DULL,
SIMPLE OR COMPLICATED,
LIBERATING OR CONFINING,
TRAGIC OR, ONCE IN A
WHILE, COMIC...

2

SEX IS A BASIC BIOLOGICAL NEED, LIKE EATING!

SEX, LIKE EATING:

* IS NECESSARY FOR THE SURVIVAL OF THE SPECIES
* FEELS GOOD
* CAUSES SLEEPINESS
* MAY BE PAINFUL IF OVERDONE
* CAN CAUSE ILLNESS
* IS SOMETIMES FOLLOWED BY SMOKING
* PROVIDES IMAGES USED IN ADVERTISING
* MAY INVOLVE PLASTIC WRAP
* CAN HAPPEN IN BED OR ON A TABLE

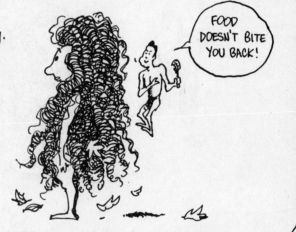

ON THE OTHER HAND...

* EATING NEVER LEADS TO PREGNANCY.
* SEX BURNS CALORIES.
* NO ONE IS TOO YOUNG TO EAT.
* EATING IS OFTEN DONE IN LARGE GROUPS.
* PEOPLE DRESS FOR DINNER.
* EATING IN PUBLIC IS O.K.
* NOBODY THINKS EATING BEFORE MARRIAGE IS SINFUL.

FOOD DOESN'T BITE YOU BACK!

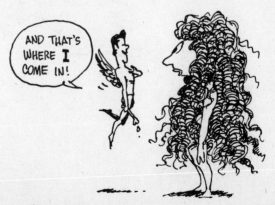

THE DIFFERENCE IS THIS: SEX (USUALLY) REQUIRES THE PARTICIPATION OF ANOTHER PERSON. THE NEGOTIATION THAT MAKES THIS HAPPEN — AND THE POTENTIAL BURDENS OF PREGNANCY — MAKE SEX A LITTLE MORE COMPLICATED THAN EATING! SEX IS BIOLOGICAL, BUT SEX IS ALSO SOCIAL.

AND THAT'S WHERE **I** COME IN!

FINALLY, ALTHOUGH SEX IS COMPLICATED, IT'S ALSO UNIVERSAL, OR NEARLY SO. 99.9% OF ALL LIVING THINGS ENGAGE IN SEX... AND IN THE NEXT CHAPTER, WE SEE WHAT, IF ANYTHING, THIS HAS TO DO WITH US!

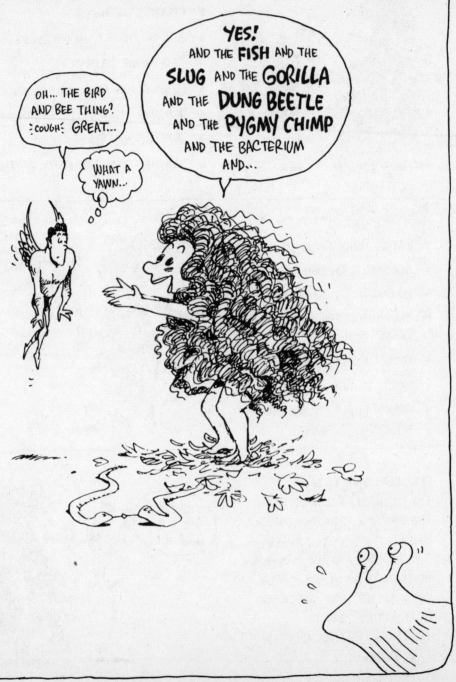

◊◊ CHAPTER 2 ◊◊

YOU'RE AN ANIMAL!
OR REPRODUCTION CAUSES SEX

Is sex really so complicated? If so, then how come nearly every plant, animal, and fungus on earth can do it? And how come people are the only ones asking any questions?

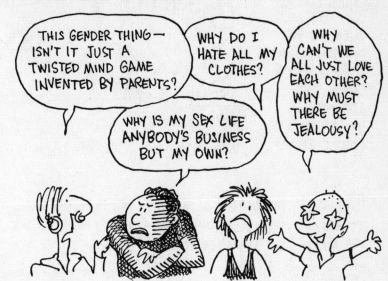

THIS GENDER THING—ISN'T IT JUST A TWISTED MIND GAME INVENTED BY PARENTS?

WHY DO I HATE ALL MY CLOTHES?

WHY CAN'T WE ALL JUST LOVE EACH OTHER? WHY MUST THERE BE JEALOUSY?

WHY IS MY SEX LIFE ANYBODY'S BUSINESS BUT MY OWN?

Maybe we can learn something about human sexuality by comparing ourselves with the rest of the natural world... so leave your preconceptions behind (but not your contraception!)... we're about to enter a place with a weird logic all its own... a place where reproduction causes sex...

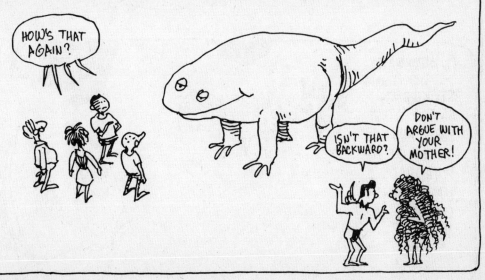

HOW'S THAT AGAIN?

ISN'T THAT BACKWARD?

DON'T ARGUE WITH YOUR MOTHER!

SEX IS EVERYWHERE. IN THE GARDEN, FLOWERS ARE JUST GARISH GENITALS THAT LURE BEES. WHEN THE BEE ARRIVES, FLOWER-SPERM RUBS OFF ON ITS LEG... AND TRAVELS BY BEE TO A FEMALE FLOWER.

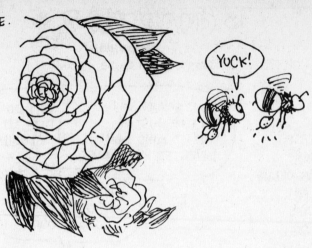

UNDERFOOT, THE GARDEN SLUG SNIFFS OUT A FELLOW SLUG... IF IT LIKES WHAT IT SMELLS, IT WILL DO ANYTHING—EVEN CHANGE ITS SEX IF NECESSARY—TO MATE WITH ITS INTENDED.

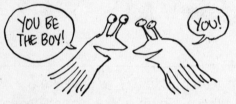

THIS CAN LEAD TO A SORT OF MATING PILE, WITH EACH SLUG A LITTLE MORE FEMALE THAN THE ONE ABOVE.

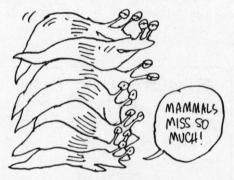

UNDERWATER, THE FEMALE STICKLEBACK LAYS A "TEST EGG" AND CHECKS OUT A POTENTIAL MATE'S NEST-GUARDING INSTINCTS.

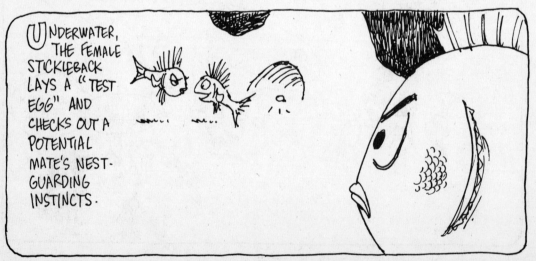

What do these examples have in common? In every case, the plant or animal is trying its hardest to

REPRODUCE SUCCESSFULLY:

Not just to reproduce, but to do so in a way that helps the offspring to survive.

REALLY? I WAS?

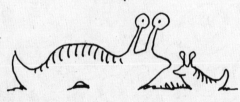

The slug, for instance, tries to sniff out a mate with "good genes," and good genes increase the offsprings' survival chances.

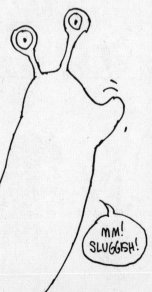

MM! SLUGGISH!

The stickleback's behavior is obviously about protecting the young.

EVEN A FISH CAN BE A STAY-AT-HOME DAD!

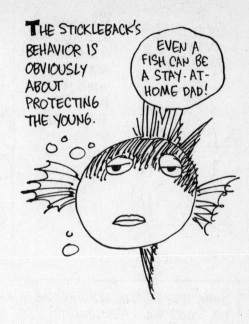

The flowering plant has a strategy, too: Since a bee tends to visit the sweetest, juiciest blossoms, high-quality sperm are likely to find high-quality eggs. In effect, flowering plants get bees to sniff out good genes for them!

PSST! BEE!

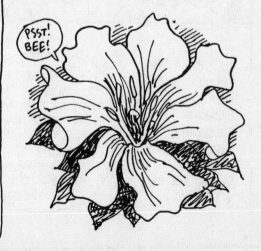

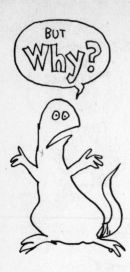

BUT
WHY?

WHY, INDEED? WHY DO PLANTS AND ANIMALS ACT THAT WAY? HERE WE ENTER THE WORLD OF WEIRD LOGIC...

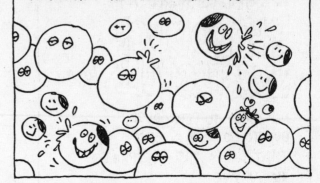

IMAGINE A POPULATION (OF ANYTHING). SOME INDIVIDUALS MAY HAVE A FEATURE (ILLUSTRATED HERE BY A BLACK SPOT) THAT HELPS THEM REPRODUCE MORE SUCCESSFULLY THAN INDIVIDUALS THAT LACK THIS FEATURE.

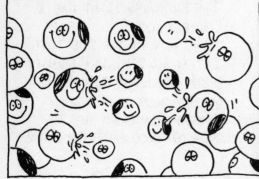

SINCE THEY REPRODUCE MORE SUCCESSFULLY, THE SUCCESSFUL TYPES COME TO OUT-NUMBER THE INCOMPETENTS AFTER SOME NUMBER OF GENERATIONS...

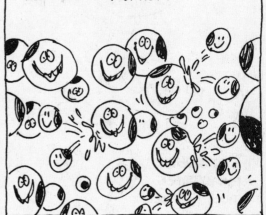

UNTIL EVENTUALLY, THEY TAKE OVER THE ENTIRE POPULATION!

IN OTHER WORDS, FEATURES AND BEHAVIORS THAT PROMOTE SUCCESSFUL REPRODUCTION TEND TO SPREAD THROUGH A POPULATION.

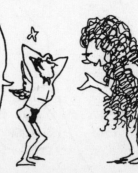

OOO... MY HEAD! YOU MEAN... EVERYONE TRIES HARD TO REPRODUCE NOW, BECAUSE EVERYONE WHO DIDN'T TRY HARD TO REPRO-DUCE DIED OUT YESTERDAY?

YUP! I CALL IT "DESIGN BY PROCESS OF ELIMINATION!"

ANOTHER EXAMPLE: ANIMALS WITH A STRONG SEX DRIVE WILL TEND TO REPRODUCE MORE THAN ANIMALS WITH A WEAK SEX DRIVE. SO NOW ALL ANIMALS HAVE A STRONG SEX DRIVE.

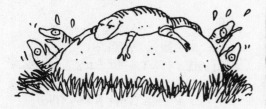

AH, BUT THEY MISS OUT ON PRECIOUS BASKING TIME!

BUT NOT TOO STRONG! HAVING SEX COMPULSIVELY CAN GET YOU IN TROUBLE, OR EVEN KILLED, WHICH CAN REALLY CUT DOWN AN ANIMAL'S ABILITY TO REPRODUCE.

YET ANOTHER EXAMPLE: WHY DOES SEX FEEL GOOD? WHY ARE SEX ORGANS WIRED WITH ALL THOSE SENSITIVE NERVE ENDINGS? SAME REASON! FEELING GOOD PROMOTES MAKING BABIES.

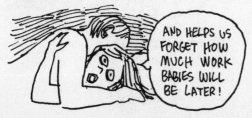

AND HELPS US FORGET HOW MUCH WORK BABIES WILL BE LATER!

Important conclusion:

IN GENERAL, JUST ABOUT EVERY ANATOMICAL FEATURE AND INSTINCTIVE BEHAVIOR IN OUR SEXUAL BIOLOGY EXISTS BECAUSE IT CONTRIBUTES TO MAKING A LOT OF LIVING OFFSPRING.

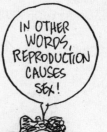

IN OTHER WORDS, REPRODUCTION CAUSES SEX!

Cautionary note:

THIS IS NOT THE SAME THING AS SAYING THAT SEX IS "FOR" REPRODUCTION. SEX CAN SERVE MANY FUNCTIONS AND RESPOND TO MANY SIGNALS, ESPECIALLY IN HUMANS. PLENTY OF SEX HAS NOTHING TO DO WITH REPRODUCTION — SAME-SEX CONTACTS BEING AN OBVIOUS EXAMPLE.

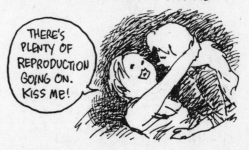

THERE'S PLENTY OF REPRODUCTION GOING ON. KISS ME!

(A LITTLE) more about genes:

HAVE YOU NOTICED SOMETHING? SO FAR, WE HAVEN'T EXACTLY SAID WHAT SEX IS... SO HERE GOES: BIOLOGICALLY, SEX IS AN EXCHANGE OF GENES.

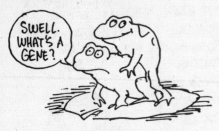

SWELL. WHAT'S A GENE?

YOU CAN THINK OF A GENE AS A KIND OF FORMULA, OR INSTRUCTION, FOR MAKING ONE OF THE BASIC CHEMICALS OF LIFE. THE FORMULA IS STORED IN THE SEQUENCE OF A LONG MOLECULE CALLED DNA →

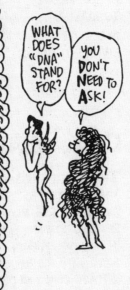

WHAT DOES "DNA" STAND FOR?

YOU DON'T NEED TO ASK!

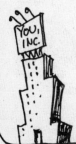

YOU, INC.

ALL YOUR GENES TAKEN TOGETHER (AROUND 100,000 OF THEM) ARE LIKE A COMPLETE BLUEPRINT FOR BUILDING.... YOU!

ALMOST EVERY CELL IN ALMOST EVERY BODY HAS TWO COMPLETE SETS OF GENES — NOT ONE, BUT TWO.

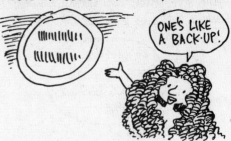

ONE'S LIKE A BACK-UP!

NATURE HAS TWO BASIC WAYS TO MAKE A NEW BODY: ONE IS TO **CLONE**: START A NEW BODY FROM A FEW CELLS OF AN OLD ONE, LIKE A PLANT RAISED FROM A CUTTING. THE CLONE HAS THE SAME GENES AS ITS PARENT.

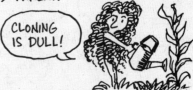

CLONING IS DULL!

THE OTHER WAY IS TO TAKE HALF THE GENES FROM ONE BODY AND HALF THE GENES FROM ANOTHER BODY.

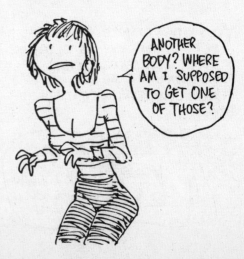

ANOTHER BODY? WHERE AM I SUPPOSED TO GET ONE OF THOSE?

H OW IS THIS
SUPPOSED TO
HAPPEN?

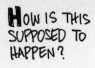
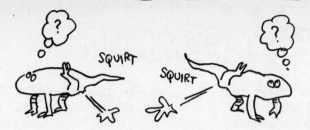

SQUIRT

SQUIRT

A BODY, BESIDES ALL ITS REGULAR CELLS, MAKES SPECIAL REPRODUCTIVE CELLS,
OR "GERM CELLS" (NOT TO BE CONFUSED WITH DISEASE-CAUSING MICROBES!).
A GERM CELL HAS ONLY ONE SET OF GENES, UNLIKE AN ORDINARY CELL,
WHICH HAS TWO:

 ORDINARY
BODY CELL

 GERM CELL

S OMEHOW, TWO GERM CELLS FROM TWO
DIFFERENT BODIES (USUALLY!) GET
TOGETHER. THAT'S FERTILIZATION.

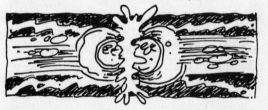

T HIS NEW, COMBINED CELL GROWS INTO A NEW BODY WITH A NEW
COMBINATION OF GENES, HALF FROM HERE AND HALF FROM THERE.

N OTE: THEY
CALL IT
"SEXUAL REPRODUCTION,"
BUT IT'S REALLY
ONLY HALF-REPRODUCTION,
SINCE EACH PARENT
GIVES UP HALF
ITS GENES IN
THE PROCESS.

SEE WHAT
WE SACRIFICE
FOR YOU?

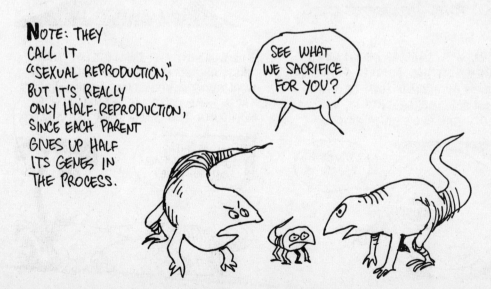

HERE'S ANOTHER LITTLE FEATURE THAT PROMOTES SUCCESSFUL REPRODUCTION:

MALE & FEMALE

ONCE UPON A TIME, LET'S IMAGINE, ALL GERM CELLS WERE ALIKE, EXCEPT THAT SOME MAY HAVE HAD SOME EXTRA NUTRIENTS AND FAT.

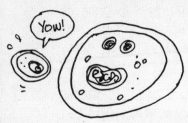

AN ENHANCED CELL, SINCE IT CARRIED ITS OWN FOOD, HAD A SURVIVAL EDGE OVER THE NON-ENHANCED.

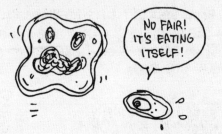

SO FAT GERM CELLS WERE WINNERS, AND EVENTUALLY HALF THE WORLD WAS MAKING THEM. WE CALL THEM **EGGS**, AND THE INDIVIDUALS THAT MAKE THEM ARE FEMALES.

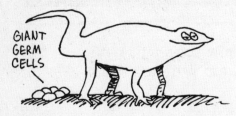

MEANWHILE, SOME OTHER INDIVIDUALS DID JUST THE OPPOSITE: THEY MADE SMALLER GERM CELLS.

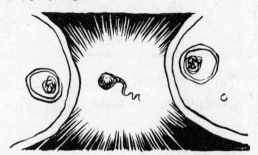

ALTHOUGH A SMALLER CELL LACKED NUTRIENTS, IT HAD ANOTHER ADVANTAGE: MOBILITY. IT COULD SWIM OR DRIFT TO AN EGG, MERGE WITH IT, AND EXPLOIT THE EGG'S NUTRIENTS.

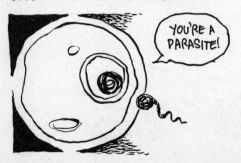

THE QUICKEST AND SMALLEST GOT THERE FIRST, AND SOON THE OTHER HALF OF THE WORLD WAS MAKING THESE MOBILE MIDGETS. THESE GERM CELLS ARE **SPERM**, AND THE INDIVIDUALS THAT MAKE THEM ARE MALES.

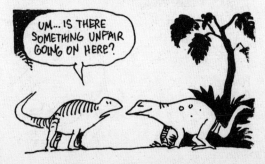

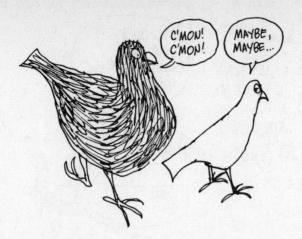

Because eggs are so much bigger than sperm, reproduction tends to be more expensive for females than for males. This makes females more cautious about choosing a mate.

All animals seek partners with good genes — or evidence of good genes, anyway, since genes are invisible — but females especially so. They may look for:

Symmetry, health, good skin, nice muscles in the right places, a caring, sensitive disposition, a brutish, insensitive disposition, or (if they're a frog) a beautiful croak.

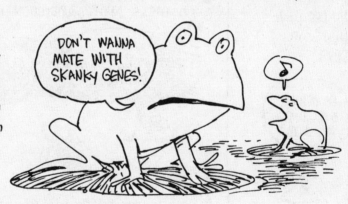

Females may also demand that the male contribute to the offsprings' well-being in other ways, like providing food. The female dung beetle, for instance, will only consider a male if he brings her a nourishing ball of dung...

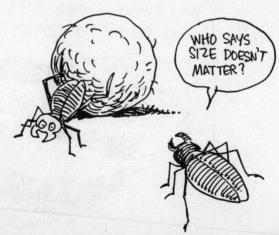

FOR MALES, ON THE OTHER HAND, REPRODUCTION IS CHEAP. WITH HIS MILLIONS OF SPERM, ONE MALE CAN THEORETICALLY HAVE FAR MORE OFFSPRING THAN ANY FEMALE. SO WHY DON'T MALES HAVE NON-STOP SEX?

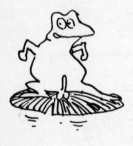

GOOD IDEA! BUT... UM... WHO WITH?

IN FACT, SOME OF THEM DO. IN A TROPICAL FISH SPECIES CALLED THE BLUEHEAD WRASSE, A FEW MALES MATE WITH 80-100 FEMALES EVERY DAY.

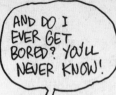

AND DO I EVER GET BORED? YOU'LL NEVER KNOW!

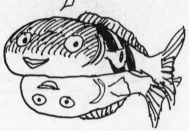

BUT MOST MALES ARE HELD BACK BY FEMALE CHOOSINESS AND COMPETITION FROM OTHER MALES.

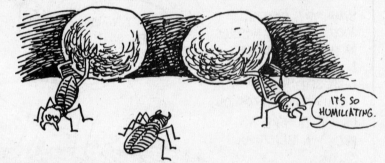

IT'S SO HUMILIATING.

AND THEN THERE ARE THE CHILDCARE DUTIES. FOR INSTANCE, THE FEMALE HORNBILL WALLS HERSELF AND THE CHICKS INTO A HOLLOW TREE, FORCING DAD TO BRING ALL THE FOOD. FOR HIM, NON-STOP SEX IS OUT OF THE QUESTION!

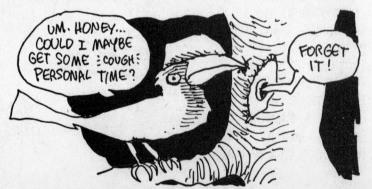

UM. HONEY... COULD I MAYBE GET SOME ᴤCOUGHᴤ PERSONAL TIME?

FORGET IT!

14

STILL, THERE'S THE ARITHMETIC: SPERM OUTNUMBER EGGS... A FEW MALES CAN IMPREGNATE MANY FEMALES...OR, TO PUT IT BLUNTLY, THERE ARE TOO MANY MALES...

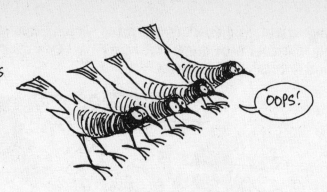

THIS EXPLAINS WHY MALES TEND TO BE MORE COMPETITIVE THAN FEMALES, AT LEAST WHEN IT COMES TO FINDING A SEX PARTNER.

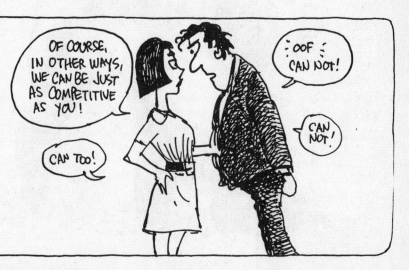

SOMETIMES, THIS COMPETITION IS PEACEFUL AND HARMLESS, LIKE THE SINGING OF MALE COWBIRDS. WHEN ONE MALE SERENADES A FEMALE, A SECOND MALE DROPS IN AND TRIES TO OUTSING HIM... THE FEMALE WATCHES ATTENTIVELY... AND SHE WILL NOT MATE WITH ANY MALE THAT OPTS OUT OF THIS COMPETITION.

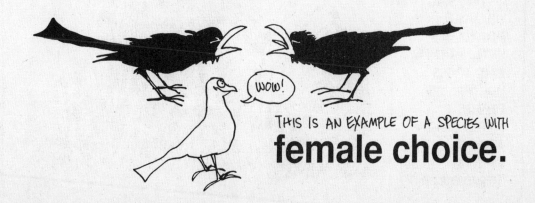

THIS IS AN EXAMPLE OF A SPECIES WITH

female choice.

AT OTHER TIMES, THE COMPETITION TURNS VIOLENT, AND MALES RISK LIFE AND LIMB BATTLING EACH OTHER FOR ACCESS TO FEMALES. DEER, CATTLE, LIONS, AND GORILLAS ARE EXAMPLES.

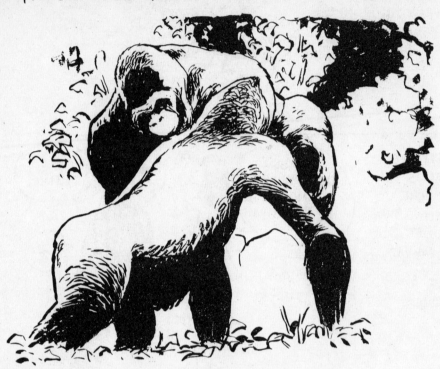

THE WINNING MALE TAKES CONTROL OF A "HAREM" OF FEMALES, WHICH HE MONOPOLIZES UNTIL ANOTHER MALE DRIVES HIM OFF. THE FEMALES HAVE LITTLE CHOICE. AFTER ALL THEY WANT TO REPRODUCE, TOO!

I NEVER MUCH LIKED MAKING DECISIONS, ANYWAY.

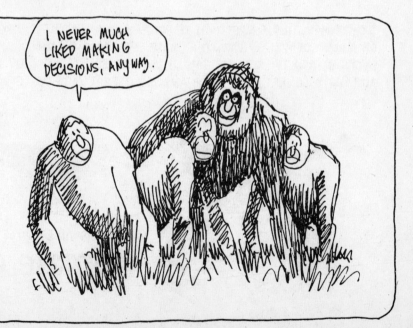

MALE COMPETITION IS MOST INTENSE WHEN ONLY A FEW MALES GET TO BREED, AND THE REST LOSE OUT.

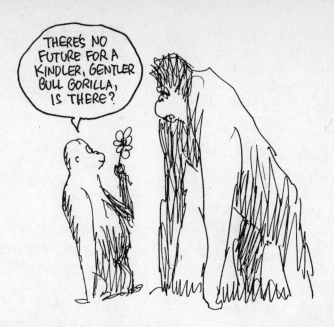

THERE'S NO FUTURE FOR A KINDLER, GENTLER BULL GORILLA, IS THERE?

WITH GORILLAS, ONLY THE VERY BIGGEST, STRONGEST, AND MOST INTIMIDATING MALES REPRODUCE... SO, IN EVERY GENERATION, THE AVERAGE MALE IS BIGGER, STRONGER, AND MORE INTIMIDATING THAN IN EARLIER GENERATIONS. BY NOW, BULL GORILLAS ARE VERY BIG, STRONG, AND FIERCE, WEIGHING ABOUT TWICE AS MUCH AS A FEMALE. THE ONLY REASON HE NEEDS THIS BULK IS PURE SEX. HE DOESN'T USE IT FOR HUNTING — GORILLAS ARE VEGETARIANS!

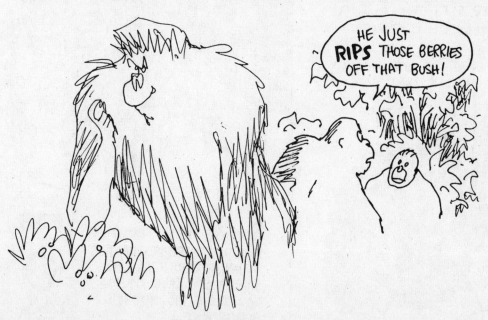

HE JUST **RIPS** THOSE BERRIES OFF THAT BUSH!

WHEN THERE IS A BIG DIFFERENCE BETWEEN MALES AND FEMALES, SCIENTISTS SAY THE SPECIES IS

SEXUALLY DIMORPHIC.

(DIMORPHIC = TWO SHAPES)

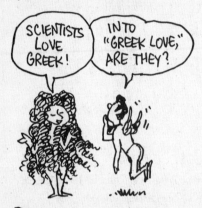

SCIENTISTS LOVE GREEK!

INTO "GREEK LOVE," ARE THEY?

SEXUAL DIMORPHISM TENDS TO GO WITH EXTREME MALE COMPETITION. WHEN ONLY A FEW MALES CAN MATE, THEY TEND TO GROW OUTLANDISH FEATURES.

OUTLANDISHLY BEAUTIFUL, THAT IS!

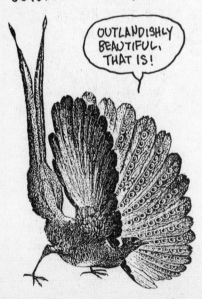

A PRIME DIMORPHIC EXAMPLE IS THE BLUEHEAD WRASSE.

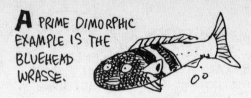

ONLY A FEW, BLUE "SUPERMALES" ARE EVER CHOSEN BY FEMALES, WHICH ARE DRAB AND TAN.

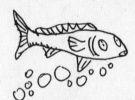

BUT THE NON-BREEDING MALES HAVE THEIR OWN DEVIOUS WAYS: THEY LOOK JUST LIKE FEMALES. WHEN A FEMALE APPROACHES A "SUPERMALE," THE DRAB MALES SWARM AROUND HER, RELEASING THEIR SPERM INTO THE WATER.

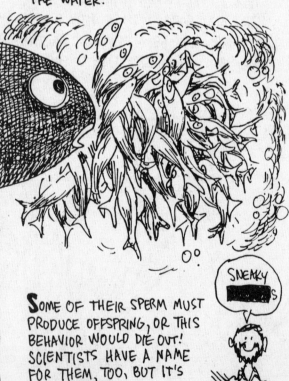

SOME OF THEIR SPERM MUST PRODUCE OFFSPRING, OR THIS BEHAVIOR WOULD DIE OUT! SCIENTISTS HAVE A NAME FOR THEM, TOO, BUT IT'S UNPRINTABLE...

SNEAKY ████S

18

SOMETIMES, ANIMALS USE PLAIN FORCE AND FRAUD...

WHEN A BULL GORILLA FIRST ACQUIRES A HAREM, HE MAY KILL ANY INFANTS FATHERED BY THE PREVIOUS MALE. DOING SO ELIMINATES COMPETING GENES AND ALSO CAUSES THE NURSING MOTHER TO BECOME FERTILE SOONER (SINCE NURSING SUPPRESSES OVULATION).

HEY! GORILLAS AREN'T THE ONLY ONES WHO ABUSE STEPCHILDREN!

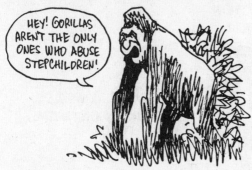

THE SHOE IS ON THE OTHER FOOT WITH THE PRAYING MANTIS. DURING THE SEX ACT, THE FEMALE MANTIS BEGINS EATING HER MATE. VERY NOURISHING FOR HER AND THE KIDS, BUT FOR HIM —?

ISN'T THAT JUST A LITTLE HARSH?

NEXT TIME I'LL JUST EAT HALF HIS HEAD.

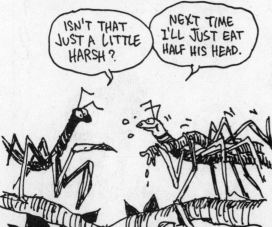

AND THEN THERE'S DECEPTION...

IN ANY CITY, YOU CAN WATCH MALE PIGEONS PUFFING THEMSELVES UP, SO FEMALES WILL THINK THEY ARE BIGGER...

OO!

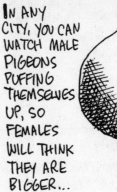
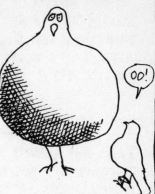

AND CHEATING: SOME MALE BIRDS KEEP A SECOND NEST, USUALLY FAR AWAY FROM THEIR MAIN RESIDENCE. THEY DIVIDE THEIR TIME BETWEEN NESTS AROUND 85-15, ENOUGH TO FATHER A FEW MORE YOUNG.

WHO CAN MEASURE LOVE?

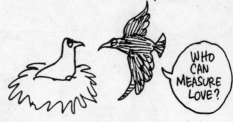

WHILE HE'S AWAY, HIS "WIFE" MAY HAVE SOME MALE VISITORS. SHE GETS TO SAMPLE SOME GENETIC VARIETY, WHILE HER LOVER FATHERS OFFSPRING TO BE RAISED AT ANOTHER'S EXPENSE.

YOUR HUSBAND IS A BIRDBRAIN!

WHERE'S YOUR WIFE?

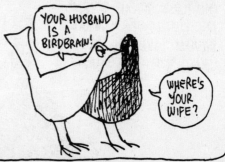

So... AS IF YOU DIDN'T KNOW IT ALREADY, SEX IS MORE THAN JUST A SIMPLE PLEASURE. IT'S WORK, AND IT'S RISKY!

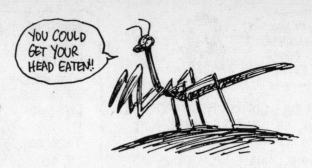

YOU COULD GET YOUR HEAD EATEN!

THAT'S WHY SO MANY ANIMALS AVOID SEX UNLESS THE FEMALE IS FERTILE — OTHERWISE, IT'S WASTED EFFORT... AND SO, IN MANY, MANY, MANY SPECIES, FEMALES SEND OUT SIGNALS THAT SAY "NOW."

FEMALE MOTHS SEND OUT CHEMICALS CALLED PHEROMONES THAT MALES CAN SMELL FROM A MILE AWAY.

FEMALE COWBIRDS STRIKE A DISTINCTIVE POSE.

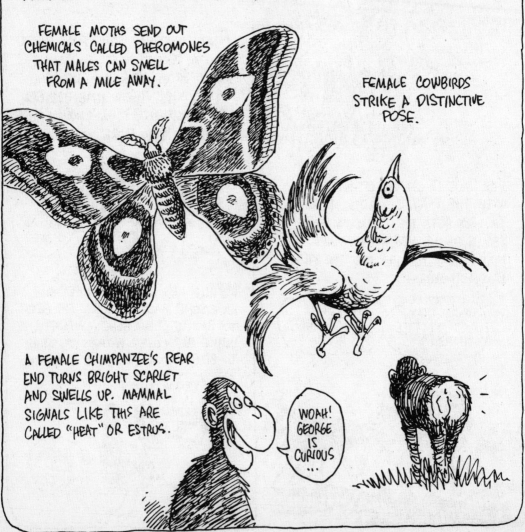

A FEMALE CHIMPANZEE'S REAR END TURNS BRIGHT SCARLET AND SWELLS UP. MAMMAL SIGNALS LIKE THIS ARE CALLED "HEAT" OR ESTRUS.

WOAH! GEORGE IS CURIOUS ...

ARE ALL ANIMALS SO... CAREFUL?

AN EXCEPTION IS THE BONOBO, A SMALL AFRICAN APE SIMILAR TO A CHIMPANZEE. BONOBOS WILL HAVE SEX AT THE DROP OF A HAT.

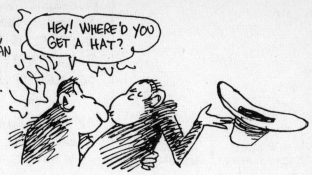

HEY! WHERE'D YOU GET A HAT?

THEY DON'T JUST HAVE SEX... THEY DO IT IN EVERY CONCEIVABLE COMBINATION: FEMALE-FEMALE, FEMALE-MALE, AND (MORE RARELY) MALE-MALE.

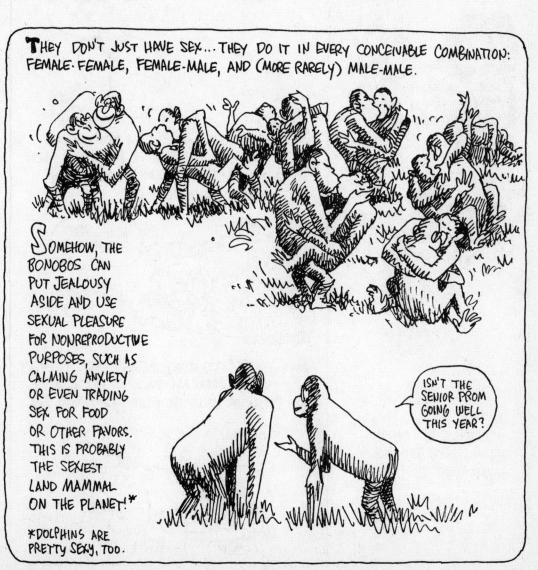

SOMEHOW, THE BONOBOS CAN PUT JEALOUSY ASIDE AND USE SEXUAL PLEASURE FOR NONREPRODUCTIVE PURPOSES, SUCH AS CALMING ANXIETY OR EVEN TRADING SEX FOR FOOD OR OTHER FAVORS. THIS IS PROBABLY THE SEXIEST LAND MAMMAL ON THE PLANET!*

*DOLPHINS ARE PRETTY SEXY, TOO.

ISN'T THE SENIOR PROM GOING WELL THIS YEAR?

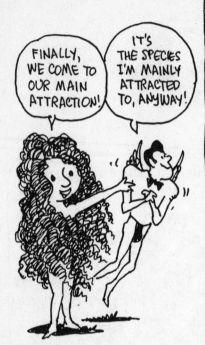

FINALLY, WE COME TO OUR MAIN ATTRACTION!

IT'S THE SPECIES I'M MAINLY ATTRACTED TO, ANYWAY!

DO WE SEE ANY ANIMAL FEATURES IN OURSELVES?

TO BEGIN WITH, THE TWO SEXES LOOK SOMEWHAT DIFFERENT. MEN, ON AVERAGE, ARE BIGGER AND STRONGER THAN WOMEN, BUT NOTHING LIKE THE DISPARITY BETWEEN MALE AND FEMALE GORILLAS.

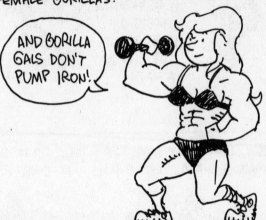

AND GORILLA GALS DON'T PUMP IRON!

THIS MODERATE DIMORPHISM GOES ALONG WITH THE FACT THAT THERE HAS LONG BEEN SOME POLYGAMY IN HUMAN SOCIETY, BUT WE'RE MAINLY MONOGAMOUS.

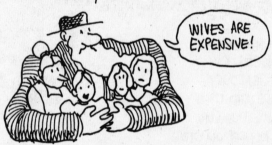

WIVES ARE EXPENSIVE!

ARE THERE "TOO MANY MALES"? UNTIL RECENTLY, ARMIES HAVE BEEN ALL-MALE, SO APPARENTLY WE CONSIDER MALES THE MORE DISPOSABLE SEX.

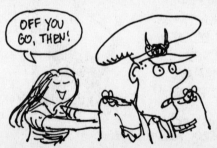

OFF YOU GO, THEN!

THERE'S NO SHORTAGE OF MALE COMPETITION: SPORTS, FOR EXAMPLE, WHERE WOMEN FLOCK TO THE TOP GUYS.

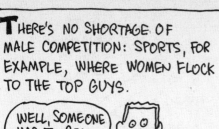

WELL, SOMEONE HAS TO READ TO ME!

OR MUSIC... THE COMPETITION IS LESS OBVIOUS, BUT THE TOP STARS DO HAVE THE MOST GROUPIES.

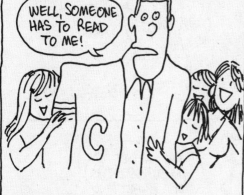

RIBBET

YES, MEN WILL COMPETE OVER NEARLY ANY- THING IN THE QUEST FOR SEX!

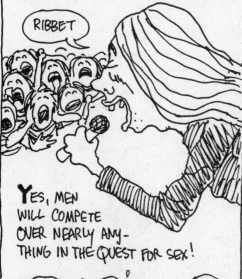

MOAN! I'M THE MOST PATHETIC!

OH, YES! YES!

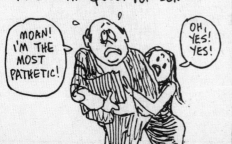

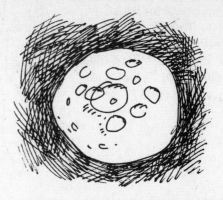

LIKE THE DUNG BEETLE, MEN WOO (OR WOW) WOMEN WITH GIFTS... ONLY WE'RE WAY AHEAD OF THE DUNG BEETLE, BECAUSE WE HAVE LANGUAGE... SO MEN CAN GIVE WOMEN SOMETHING NO BEETLE COULD DREAM OF: PROMISES.

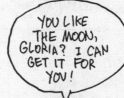

YOU LIKE THE MOON, GLORIA? I CAN GET IT FOR YOU!

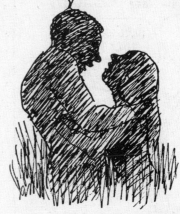

HOW ABOUT OUR DIFFERENCES FROM OTHER ANIMALS? WELL, THERE'S ALWAYS UPRIGHT POSTURE. WHEN WE STOOD UP, "BACK THERE" TURNED INTO "DOWN THERE." THIS WAS CONFUSING!

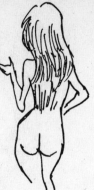

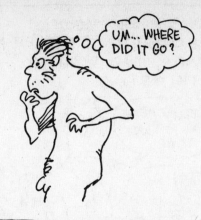

UM... WHERE DID IT GO?

HOW WAS A MALE SUPPOSED TO SEE THE SWOLLEN, FIRE-ENGINE-RED SEX ORGANS THAT SIGNALED A FEMALE IN ESTRUS?

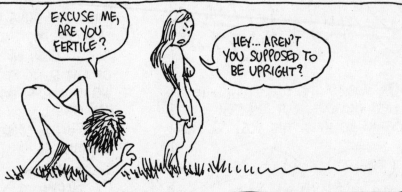

EXCUSE ME, ARE YOU FERTILE?

HEY... AREN'T YOU SUPPOSED TO BE UPRIGHT?

NOT ONLY THAT, BUT THE OLD SEXUAL POSITIONS DIDN'T WORK AS WELL AS THEY USED TO.

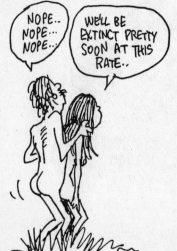

NOPE.. NOPE... NOPE...

WE'LL BE EXTINCT PRETTY SOON AT THIS RATE..

WELL... WE DID SOLVE THAT PROBLEM (SEE CHAPTER 7)... BUT IT SEEMS THE HUMAN MALE STILL HAS A TROUBLESOME "FOSSIL RESPONSE" TO THE FEMALE POSTERIOR.

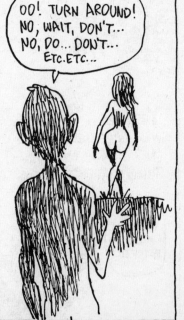

OO! TURN AROUND! NO, WAIT, DON'T... NO, DO... DON'T... ETC. ETC...

24

HERE'S ANOTHER DIFFERENCE: AT SOME POINT IN HISTORY, HUMAN FEMALES STOPPED HAVING SWOLLEN, FIRE-ENGINE-RED SEX ORGANS DURING FERTILE PERIODS. WE HAVE NO ESTRUS — WOMEN CONCEAL THEIR FERTILITY.

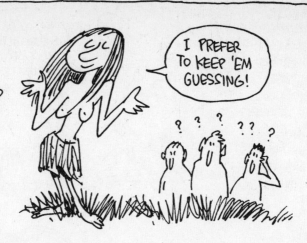

I PREFER TO KEEP 'EM GUESSING!

THIS IS VERY UNUSUAL. UNLIKE "NORMAL" MAMMALS, WOMEN CAN BE SEXUALLY RECEPTIVE WITHOUT BEING FERTILE.

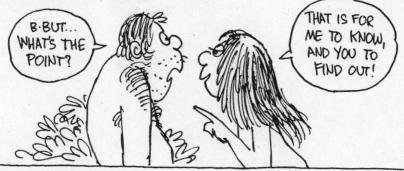

B-BUT... WHAT'S THE POINT?

THAT IS FOR ME TO KNOW, AND YOU TO FIND OUT!

MEN, MEANWHILE, NATURALLY LEARNED TO RESPOND TO SEXUAL SIGNALS, NOT FERTILITY SIGNALS. THE MERE SHAPE OF WOMEN SETS MEN OFF!

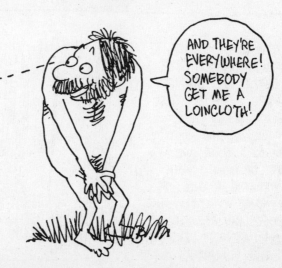

AND THEY'RE EVERYWHERE! SOMEBODY GET ME A LOINCLOTH!

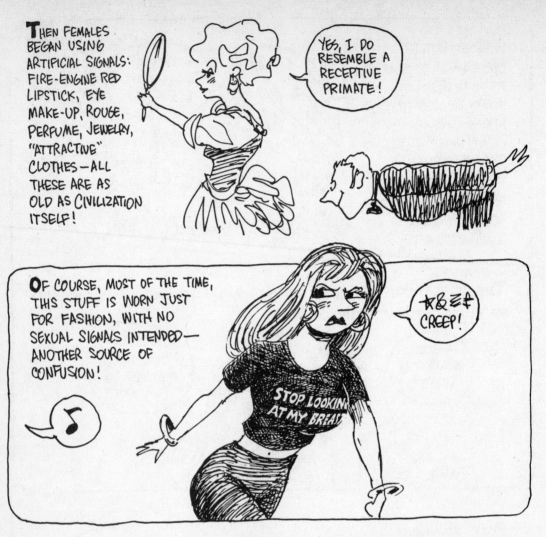

THEN FEMALES BEGAN USING ARTIFICIAL SIGNALS: FIRE-ENGINE RED LIPSTICK, EYE MAKE-UP, ROUGE, PERFUME, JEWELRY, "ATTRACTIVE" CLOTHES—ALL THESE ARE AS OLD AS CIVILIZATION ITSELF!

YES, I DO RESEMBLE A RECEPTIVE PRIMATE!

OF COURSE, MOST OF THE TIME, THIS STUFF IS WORN JUST FOR FASHION, WITH NO SEXUAL SIGNALS INTENDED—ANOTHER SOURCE OF CONFUSION!

*&≠£ CREEP!

STOP LOOKING AT MY BREASTS

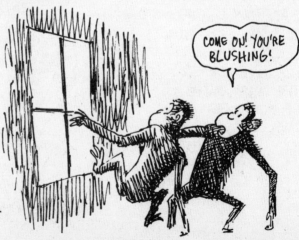

PUT IT ALL TOGETHER, AND WHAT DO YOU GET? A VERY FLUID SEXUALITY: WE ARE A SPECIES THAT CAN DO IT ANY TIME, ANYWHERE, AND ANY WAY... ONE AT A TIME, TWO AT A TIME, OR MORE... WITH A VIBRATOR, A SHOE, OR YOU NAME IT... AFTER THE BONOBOS, WE ARE THE SECOND-SEXIEST LAND MAMMAL ON THE PLANET!!

COME ON! YOU'RE BLUSHING!

26

A THIRD BIG DIFFERENCE IS OUR BRAINS, WHICH ARE BIG AND COMPLICATED. WE'RE THE SMART SPECIES!

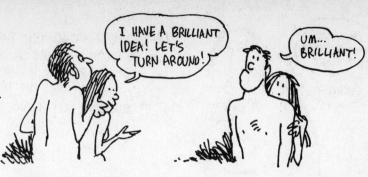

THESE BIG BRAINS ARE SLOW TO FILL UP... HUMANS TAKE A LONG TIME TO MATURE... AND KIDS DO BETTER WHEN THEY HAVE GUIDANCE AND SUPPORT FROM BOTH PARENTS FOR A VERY LONG TIME... AND SO WE FORM COUPLES AND FAMILIES.

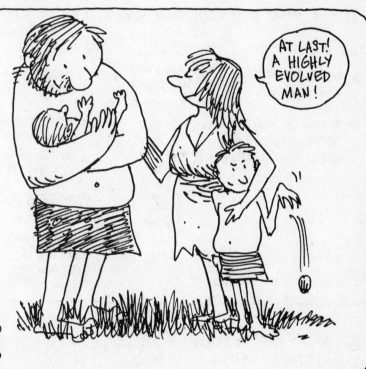

ONE THEORY SUGGESTS THAT THE LOSS OF ESTRUS HOLDS FAMILIES TOGETHER. BY BEING SEXUALLY ACCESSIBLE, WOMEN KEEP THEIR MATES NEARBY, AND BY HIDING FERTILITY, THEY KEEP THEM GUESSING!

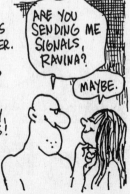

THE POINT IS THAT WE HAVE SOME BUILT-IN FEATURES THAT DRAW US INTO LONG-TERM RELATIONSHIPS AND KEEP US THERE.

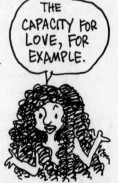

27

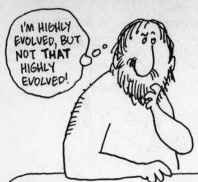

I'M HIGHLY EVOLVED, BUT NOT **THAT** HIGHLY EVOLVED!

ONE THING ABOUT ALL THAT PARENTING: IF A MAN HAS TO SPEND 15 YEARS OR SO RAISING A CHILD, HE WANTS TO BE FAIRLY CERTAIN THAT HE IS REALLY THE FATHER. THE BIOLOGICAL PAYOFF IS REPRODUCTION, NOT BEING A NICE GUY!

THAT IS, MALES AND FEMALES HAVE SLIGHTLY DIFFERENT REPRODUCTIVE AGENDAS:

SHE WANTS:

* DESIRABLE SEXUAL PARTNERS

* A MAN OR MEN AROUND TO HELP FEED AND RAISE THE CHILDREN.

COMPLETELY REASONABLE.

HE WANTS:

* DESIRABLE SEXUAL PARTNERS

* A WOMAN OR WOMEN TO BEAR HIS CHILDREN AND HELP RAISE AND FEED THEM

PLUS:

* THE ASSURANCE THAT THOSE CHILDREN ARE REALLY HIS!

WITHOUT DNA TESTING, HOW AM I SUPPOSED TO KNOW?

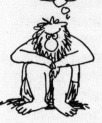

AND SO, ALL OVER THE WORLD, COUPLES STRIKE A DEAL: A **PROMISE** OF MUTUAL SUPPORT AND FIDELITY.* IN OTHER WORDS, THEY GET MARRIED.

YOU MAY NOW DO IT LEGALLY.

(*EXCEPT IN POLYGAMOUS SOCIETIES, WHERE HUSBANDS GET TO MONOPOLIZE THEIR WIVES' GENES, BUT NOT VICE VERSA.)

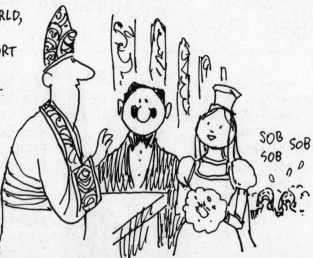

SOB SOB SOB

28

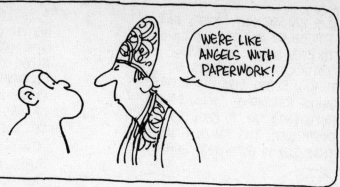

MARRIAGE IS A CULTURAL WAY OF SOLVING A BIOLOGICAL PROBLEM. PEOPLE ARE THE ONLY ANIMALS THAT CAN SWEAR VOWS, TAKE BLOOD TESTS, FILE THEIR TAXES JOINTLY, ETC.

WE'RE LIKE ANGELS WITH PAPERWORK!

THE INSTITUTION OF MARRIAGE HAS HELD UP PRETTY WELL OVER THE YEARS, BUT THERE ARE A COUPLE OF PROBLEMS.

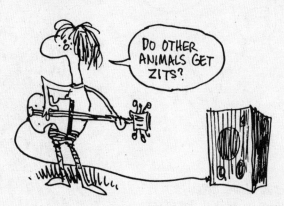

CULTURE HAS RACED AHEAD OF BIOLOGY. BIOLOGICALLY, WE CAN BREED BY THE AGE OF ABOUT 13, LONG BEFORE WE ARE READY FOR ANY LONG·TERM COMMITMENTS. AND SO WE HAVE A LONG, PAINFUL ADOLESCENCE.

DO OTHER ANIMALS GET ZITS?

THEN, WHEN WE DO ENTER A RELATIONSHIP, WE PLEDGE OURSELVES TO ONLY ONE — AND MEANWHILE, WE ARE THE SECOND-SEXIEST LAND MAMMAL ON THE PLANET!!

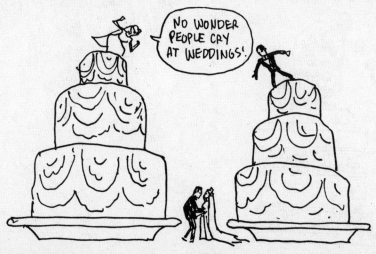

NO WONDER PEOPLE CRY AT WEDDINGS!

DO YOU SEE WHY SOCIETY HAS STRUGGLED SO LONG AND HARD TO KEEP SEXUALITY UNDER CONTROL? GOVERNMENTS TRY TO BAN SEXUAL "IRREGULARITIES," WHILE RELIGIONS (WELL, SOME RELIGIONS) TRY TO COOL US DOWN WITH THE AMUSING IDEA THAT SEX IS DIRTY AND SINFUL.

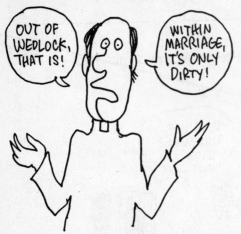

OUT OF WEDLOCK, THAT IS!

WITHIN MARRIAGE, IT'S ONLY DIRTY!

OUR THINKERS HAVE INVENTED SUCH CONCEPTS AS HONOR, FIDELITY, CHASTITY, PROMISCUITY, RESPONSIBILITY, CHIVALRY, RESPECT, MODESTY, DECENCY, PROPRIETY...

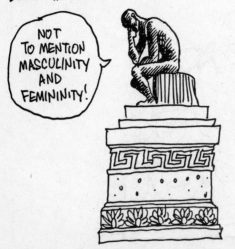

NOT TO MENTION MASCULINITY AND FEMININITY!

OUR LEADERS HAVE CREATED INSTITUTIONS AND REGULATIONS LIKE THE TEN COMMANDMENTS, BLOOD TESTS, MARRIAGE LICENSES, INCOME TAX PENALTIES, DATING RITUALS, DANCES, AN AGE OF CONSENT, DRESS CODES, DOWRIES, DIVORCE COURTS, ALIMONY, CHILD-SUPPORT LAWS, DOMESTIC PARTNERSHIP, COMMUNITY PROPERTY...

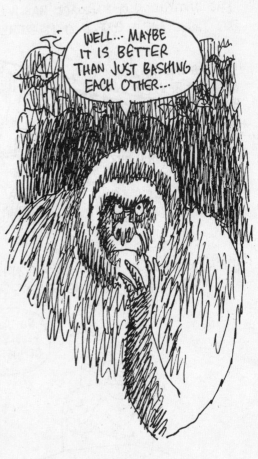

WELL... MAYBE IT IS BETTER THAN JUST BASHING EACH OTHER...

MUCH OF THAT LOAD OF CONCEPTS AND CUSTOMS IS ESPECIALLY DESIGNED TO CONTROL FEMALE SEXUALITY IN PARTICULAR.

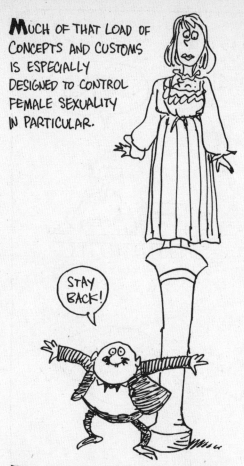

STAY BACK!

TAKE THE CONCEPT OF A WOMAN'S HONOR... IT JUST MEANS HER GENETIC PURITY, AND IT SPRINGS FROM THE MALE'S DESIRE TO MONOPOLIZE HIS MATE'S GENES. A WOMAN'S HONOR IS SUPPOSED TO BE SPOTLESS, LIKE BRAND-NEW UNDERWEAR.

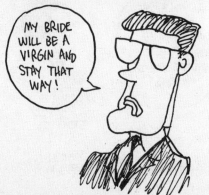

MY BRIDE WILL BE A VIRGIN AND STAY THAT WAY!

IN THEIR ZEAL TO CONTROL FEMALE SEXUALITY, THE MALES OF MANY SOCIETIES, BOTH EASTERN AND WESTERN, HAVE TRIED TO CONTROL EVERYTHING ELSE ABOUT WOMEN, TOO.

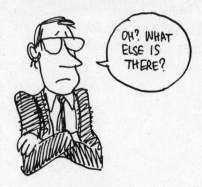

OH? WHAT ELSE IS THERE?

WOMEN HAVE FACED RESTRICTIONS ON OWNING PROPERTY, WORKING OUTSIDE THE HOME, OR HAVING ANY ROLE IN GOVERNMENT. IN SOME PLACES, WOMEN HAVE BEEN REGARDED AS THE PROPERTY OF MEN. THIS WHOLE, LOPSIDED SITUATION IS CALLED

PATRIARCHY*

("FATHERS RULE").

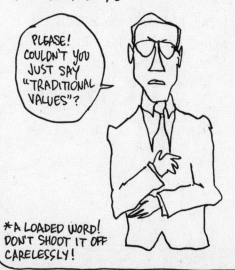

PLEASE! COULDN'T YOU JUST SAY "TRADITIONAL VALUES"?

*A LOADED WORD! DON'T SHOOT IT OFF CARELESSLY!

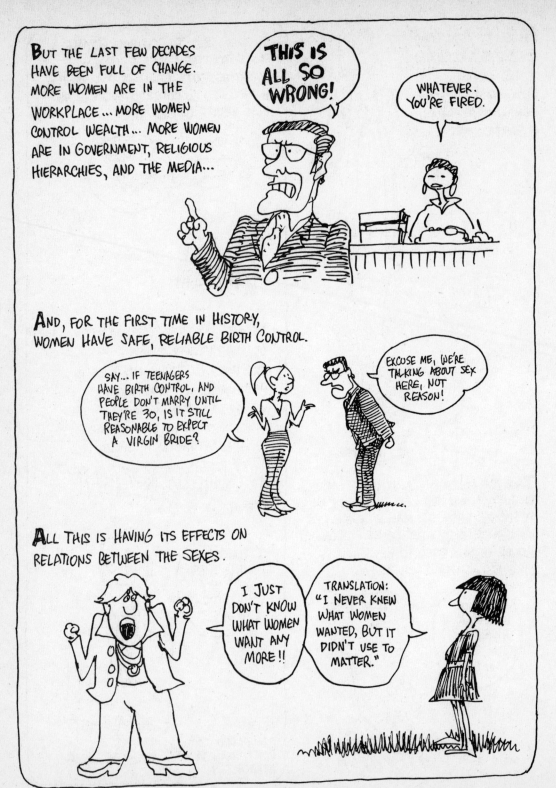

IT HAS ALSO RAISED QUESTIONS ABOUT THE MEANING OR PURPOSE OF SEX ITSELF. IF WE CAN CONTROL OUR REPRODUCTION, WHAT IS SEX "FOR" OR "ABOUT" MOST OF THE TIME?

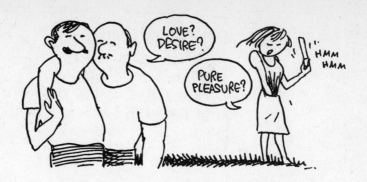

AS TRADITIONAL VALUES HAVE CRUMBLED, WE'VE ALSO SEEN A RISE IN TEEN PREGNANCY AND AN EPIDEMIC OF SEXUALLY TRANSMISSIBLE DISEASES.

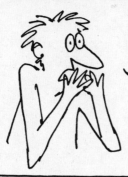

WE MAY HAVE TO DO THE UNTHINKABLE: DISCUSS SEX OPENLY AND REALISTICALLY!

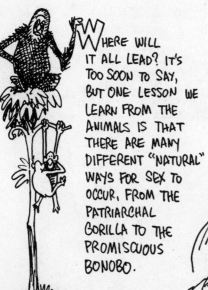

WHERE WILL IT ALL LEAD? IT'S TOO SOON TO SAY, BUT ONE LESSON WE LEARN FROM THE ANIMALS IS THAT THERE ARE MANY DIFFERENT "NATURAL" WAYS FOR SEX TO OCCUR, FROM THE PATRIARCHAL GORILLA TO THE PROMISCUOUS BONOBO.

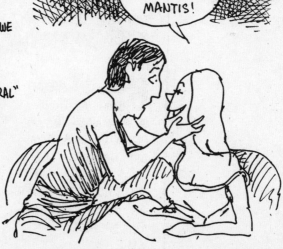

AND DON'T FORGET THE PRAYING MANTIS!

FOR THE TIME BEING, LET'S SEE IF WE'RE ANY CLOSER TO ANSWERING THE QUESTIONS AT THE TOP OF THE CHAPTER.

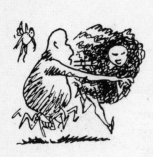

SOCIETY'S INVOLVEMENT WITH SEXUALITY? IT LOOKS PRETTY NATURAL, DESPITE WHAT MANY OF US MIGHT HOPE!

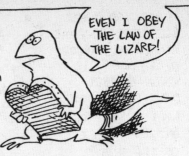

EVEN I OBEY THE LAW OF THE LIZARD!

JEALOUSY? SOME OF IT IS INSTINCTIVE, CERTAINLY. HOW WE EXPRESS OUR JEALOUSY IS SOCIALLY REGULATED, THOUGH.

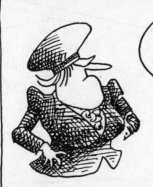

THIS SOCIETY FROWNS ON HOMICIDAL RAGES!

CLOTHES? A WAY TO CONCEAL SEXUALITY... A WAY TO FLAUNT SEXUALITY... A WAY TO KEEP WARM.

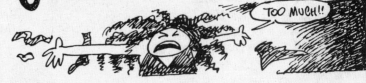

TOO MUCH!!

GENDER? SOME OF WHAT WE THINK OF AS MASCULINE AND FEMININE IS A SOCIAL ARRANGEMENT. ON THE OTHER HAND, IF YOU STILL HAVE DOUBTS ABOUT OUR BIOLOGICAL DIFFERENCES, READ ON...

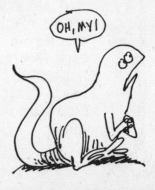

OH, MY!

· CHAPTER 3 ·

HUMAN SEXUAL ANATOMY, OR A HANDBOOK FOR AMATEUR PLUMBERS

When you think about it, the two sexes are really pretty similar. Almost all of us are born with arms, legs, ears, eyes, and lungs, plus a heart, a liver, a brain, a nose...

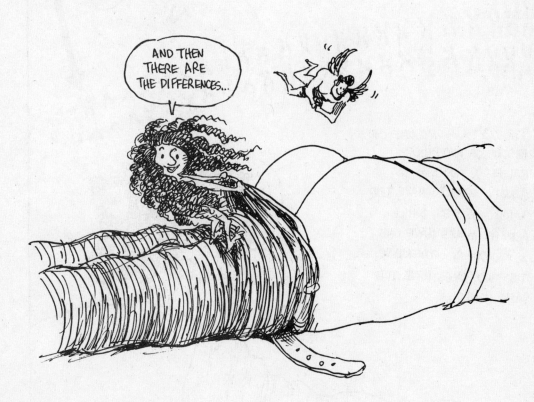

AND THEN THERE ARE THE DIFFERENCES...

OUR SIMILARITIES BEGIN IN OUR GENES.
MALES AND FEMALES BOTH HAVE 23
PAIRS OF CHROMOSOMES, OR GENE CLUSTERS,
AND OUT OF ALL THOSE, ONLY TWO MAKE
A SEXUAL DIFFERENCE: PAIR #23.

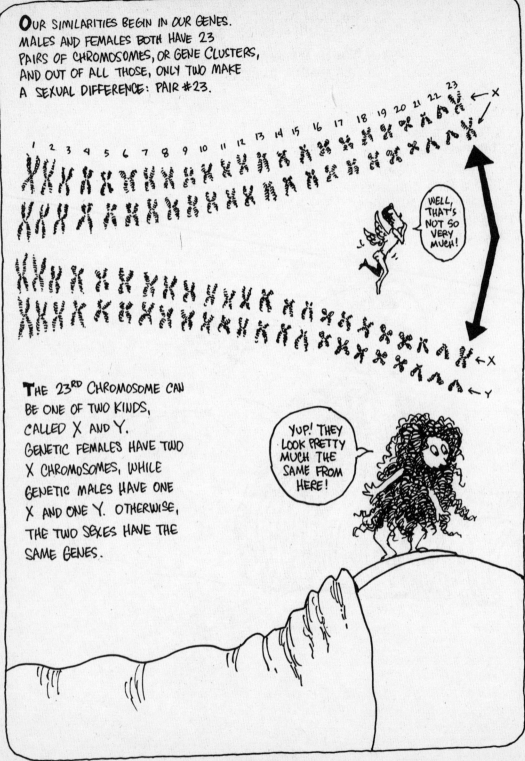

WELL, THAT'S NOT SO VERY MUCH!

THE 23RD CHROMOSOME CAN
BE ONE OF TWO KINDS,
CALLED X AND Y.
GENETIC FEMALES HAVE TWO
X CHROMOSOMES, WHILE
GENETIC MALES HAVE ONE
X AND ONE Y. OTHERWISE,
THE TWO SEXES HAVE THE
SAME GENES.

YUP! THEY LOOK PRETTY MUCH THE SAME FROM HERE!

WHEN A FEMALE MAKES EGGS, EVERY EGG GETS AN X.

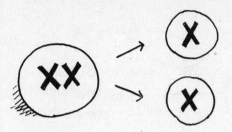

WHEN A MALE MAKES SPERM, HALF GET X AND HALF GET Y.

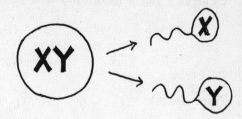

FERTILIZATION THEN THEORETICALLY MAKES HALF MALES AND HALF FEMALES:

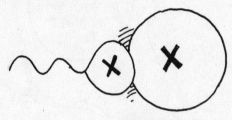

FEMALE

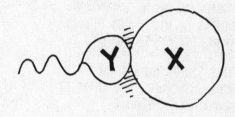

MALE

NOTE: FOR A VARIETY OF REASONS, THINGS AREN'T ALWAYS SO SIMPLE. SOMETIMES SPERM MAKES MISTAKES SORTING OUT CHROMOSOMES. WHEN THESE MEET EGGS, THEY CREATE UNUSUAL GENETIC COMBINATIONS LIKE XXY AND X ALONE.

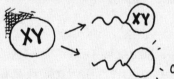

NO SEX CHROMOSOME

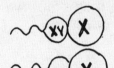

XXY = "KLINEFELTER'S SYNDROME"

X = "TURNER'S FEMALE"

EVEN UNDER NORMAL CONDITIONS, SPERM WITH X ARE A LITTLE HEAVIER THAN SPERM WITH Y... SOMETIMES EGGS SEEM TO FAVOR ONE KIND OF SPERM OR THE OTHER... AND MALE EMBRYOS SPONTANEOUSLY FALL MORE OFTEN THAN FEMALES... RESULT: CONCEPTIONS ARE MORE THAN 50% MALE, BUT BIRTHS ARE MORE THAN 50% FEMALE.

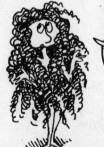

OH, WELL, NOBODY'S PERFECT!

EVERYBODY HAS AN X CHROMOSOME. THIS MAY EXPLAIN WHY ALL EMBRYOS DEVELOP IN EXACTLY THE SAME WAY AT FIRST. BY SIX WEEKS AFTER CONCEPTION, SEX ORGANS ARE THE SAME IN EVERYONE: JUST A GROOVE AND SOME SWELLING.

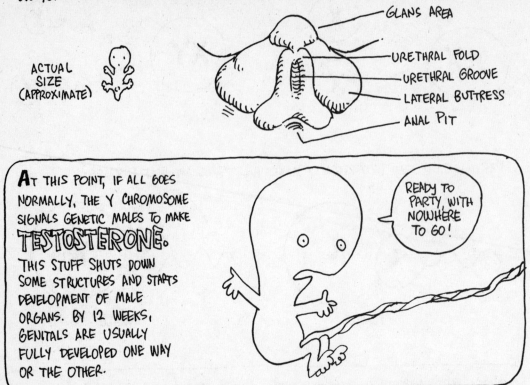

ACTUAL SIZE (APPROXIMATE)

- GLANS AREA
- URETHRAL FOLD
- URETHRAL GROOVE
- LATERAL BUTTRESS
- ANAL PIT

AT THIS POINT, IF ALL GOES NORMALLY, THE Y CHROMOSOME SIGNALS GENETIC MALES TO MAKE **TESTOSTERONE.** THIS STUFF SHUTS DOWN SOME STRUCTURES AND STARTS DEVELOPMENT OF MALE ORGANS. BY 12 WEEKS, GENITALS ARE USUALLY FULLY DEVELOPED ONE WAY OR THE OTHER.

READY TO PARTY, WITH NOWHERE TO GO!

AROUND 1-2% OF THE TIME, GENETIC OR HORMONAL FACTORS PRODUCE BABIES THAT ARE NOT EXACTLY ONE OR THE OTHER. THEY MAY HAVE VERY SMALL MALE GENITALS, AMBIGUOUS GENITALS, OR TWO SETS OF GENITALS.

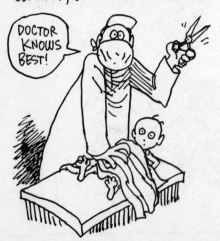

DOCTOR KNOWS BEST!

UNTIL RECENTLY, SURGEONS RUSHED TO "FIX" THESE CHILDREN TO MAKE THEM LOOK FEMALE. THIS PRACTICE IS NOW BEING QUESTIONED BY SOME OF ITS VICTIMS, WHO HAVE BECOME "AMBIGUITY ADVOCATES."

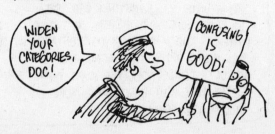

WIDEN YOUR CATEGORIES, DOC!

CONFUSING IS GOOD!

BECAUSE OF THEIR ROLE IN REPRODUCTION, THE SEX ORGANS OF BOTH MALES AND FEMALES ARE SOMETIMES CALLED

GENITALS,

FROM LATIN GENERE, MEANING TO BEGET OR GENERATE. THEY HAVE SOME OTHER NAMES, TOO...

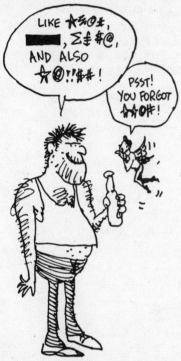

LIKE ✳︎☀︎◎✣, ▬, Σ✢ $@, AND ALSO ✩◎‼︎✱✣!

PSST! YOU FORGOT ✩◎✣!

AND THEY HAVE ANOTHER ROLE, TOO: BECAUSE OF THE MUTUAL PLEASURE THAT SEX PARTNERS GIVE EACH OTHER, SEX ORGANS HELP CREATE AND MAINTAIN HUMAN RELATIONSHIPS.

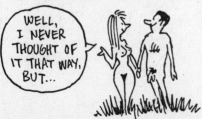

WELL, I NEVER THOUGHT OF IT THAT WAY, BUT...

THEY'RE SO IMPORTANT, IN FACT, THAT UNLIKE OTHER ANIMALS, WE KEEP THEM UNDER WRAPS, EXCEPT ON SPECIAL OCCASIONS... AND SO GENITALS HAVE COME TO SEEM MYSTERIOUS, SCARY, AND DANGEROUS.

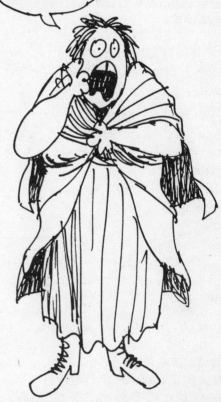

CIVILIZATION IS DOOMED UNLESS WE COVER OUR WEEWEES!

(ONE 18TH-CENTURY EDUCATOR RECOMMENDED TEACHING CHILDREN ABOUT SEXUAL ANATOMY BY SHOWING THEM CORPSES, WHICH, HE REASONED, WOULD KEEP THE STUDENTS IN A PROPERLY SOBER FRAME OF MIND. IN THIS BOOK, WE'LL USE LINE DRAWINGS...)

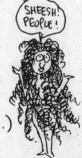

SHEESH! PEOPLE!

IN BOTH SEXES, EXTERNAL ORGANS ARE CONNECTED TO INTERNAL ONES. HERE IS THE **VULVA,** AS THE GROUP OF EXTERNAL ORGANS IS CALLED. THE VULVA'S SENSITIVE AND/OR PROTECTIVE STRUCTURES SURROUND THE VAGINAL OPENING, WHICH LEADS TO THE UTERUS (SEE P. 42).

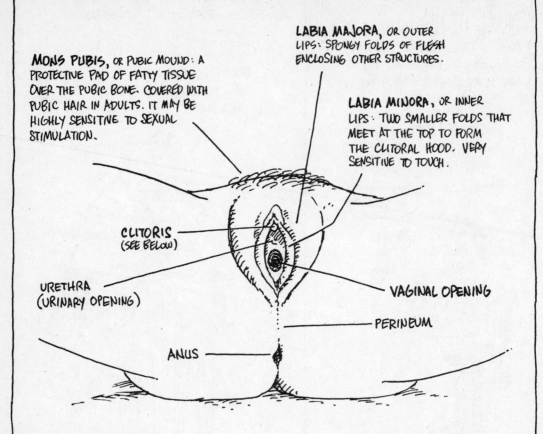

MONS PUBIS, OR PUBIC MOUND: A PROTECTIVE PAD OF FATTY TISSUE OVER THE PUBIC BONE. COVERED WITH PUBIC HAIR IN ADULTS. IT MAY BE HIGHLY SENSITIVE TO SEXUAL STIMULATION.

LABIA MAJORA, OR OUTER LIPS: SPONGY FOLDS OF FLESH ENCLOSING OTHER STRUCTURES.

LABIA MINORA, OR INNER LIPS: TWO SMALLER FOLDS THAT MEET AT THE TOP TO FORM THE CLITORAL HOOD. VERY SENSITIVE TO TOUCH.

CLITORIS (SEE BELOW)

URETHRA (URINARY OPENING)

VAGINAL OPENING

PERINEUM

ANUS

THE CLITORIS, LOADED WITH NERVE ENDINGS, IS THE FOCUS OF FEMALE SEXUAL AROUSAL. ONLY THE TIP OR GLANS IS VISIBLE, BUT THE SHAFT CONTINUES UNDER THE CLITORAL HOOD AND HAS TWO SIDE BRANCHES CALLED CRURA. WHEN STIMULATED, THE WHOLE CLITORIS CAN BECOME ENGORGED WITH BLOOD. IT IS THE ONLY ORGAN IN EITHER SEX WHOSE SOLE FUNCTION IS SEXUAL AROUSAL.

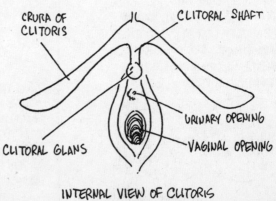

CRURA OF CLITORIS

CLITORAL SHAFT

URINARY OPENING

VAGINAL OPENING

CLITORAL GLANS

INTERNAL VIEW OF CLITORIS

AT BIRTH, THE VAGINAL OPENING IS PARTLY COVERED BY A THIN MEMBRANE OF SKIN CALLED THE HYMEN (AFTER THE ROMAN GOD OF MARRIAGE). THE HYMEN IS PERFORATED, ALLOWING MENSTRUAL BLOOD AND VAGINAL SECRETIONS TO PASS OUT OF THE BODY.

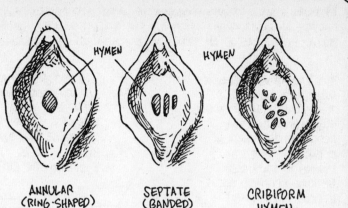

ANNULAR (RING-SHAPED) HYMEN

SEPTATE (BANDED) HYMEN

CRIBIFORM HYMEN

THE HYMEN CAN BE STRETCHED OR TORN IN MANY WAYS: INSERTION OF TAMPONS, MANUAL SEX PLAY, SEXUAL INTERCOURSE, OR THE PROVERBIAL BICYCLE ACCIDENT.

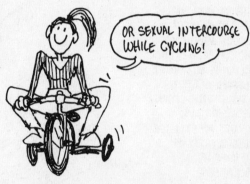

OR SEXUAL INTERCOURSE WHILE CYCLING!

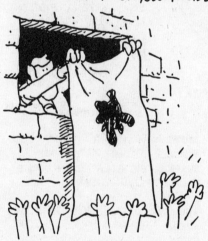

IN MANY CULTURES, PAST AND PRESENT, AN INTACT HYMEN IS AN ESSENTIAL ITEM FOR A BRIDE. THE BLOOD-STAINED SHEET MAY EVEN BE DISPLAYED TO CHEERING RELATIVES AFTER THE WEDDING NIGHT AS PROOF OF THE BRIDE'S HONOR.

IN SOME OF THOSE PLACES, THERE IS A HIGH DEMAND FOR PLASTIC SURGEONS — TO RECONSTRUCT THE HYMENS OF BRIDES-TO-BE.

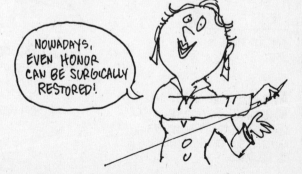

NOWADAYS, EVEN HONOR CAN BE SURGICALLY RESTORED!

INTERNAL FEMALE ORGANS PRODUCE EGGS, OFFER A CHANNEL FOR SPERM TO REACH THE EGG, AND PROVIDE AN ENVIRONMENT WHERE THE FERTILIZED EGG CAN DIVIDE, DEVELOP, AND GROW. EGG PRODUCTION RUNS ON AN APPROXIMATELY MONTHLY CYCLE, REGULATED BY HORMONES.

THE VAGINA IS A FLEXIBLE, MUSCULAR TUBE, ABOUT 3-4 INCHES LONG IN ADULTS. THE VAGINA HAS TWO REPRODUCTIVE FUNCTIONS: IT ENCLOSES THE PENIS DURING INTERCOURSE, BRINGING SPERM TO THE UTERUS, AND IT IS THE BIRTH CANAL THROUGH WHICH AN INFANT IS BORN.

THE VAGINAL WALLS ARE LINED WITH MUCOUS MEMBRANES THAT SECRETE FLUIDS, INCLUDING LUBRICANTS RELEASED IN RESPONSE TO SEXUAL STIMULATION. THE VAGINA ALSO PROVIDES AN EXIT FOR THESE SECRETIONS AND UTERINE DISCHARGES.

THE UTERUS (OR WOMB) IS A HOLLOW, THICK-WALLED ORGAN THAT HOLDS THE FETUS DURING PREGNANCY, WHEN THE UTERUS MAY EXPAND TO THE SIZE OF A VOLLEYBALL OR LARGER. THE UTERINE LINING, OR ENDOMETRIUM, IS FILLED WITH BLOOD VESSELS. THE OPENING OF THE UTERUS IS CALLED THE CERVIX.

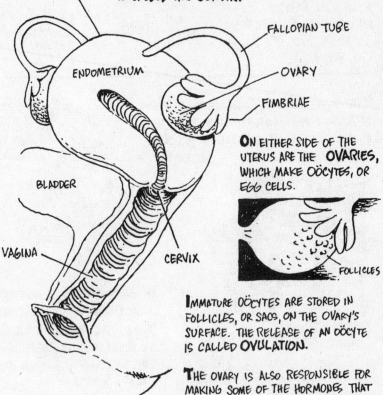

UTERUS

FALLOPIAN TUBE

ENDOMETRIUM

OVARY

FIMBRIAE

BLADDER

VAGINA

CERVIX

ON EITHER SIDE OF THE UTERUS ARE THE OVARIES, WHICH MAKE OÖCYTES, OR EGG CELLS.

FOLLICLES

IMMATURE OÖCYTES ARE STORED IN FOLLICLES, OR SACS, ON THE OVARY'S SURFACE. THE RELEASE OF AN OÖCYTE IS CALLED OVULATION.

THE OVARY IS ALSO RESPONSIBLE FOR MAKING SOME OF THE HORMONES THAT REGULATE THE REPRODUCTIVE CYCLE.

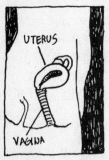

UTERUS

VAGINA

ORIENTATION IN BODY

FALLOPIAN TUBES CONVEY THE OÖCYTE FROM THE OVARY TO THE UTERUS. THE FALLOPIAN TUBES DO NOT TOUCH THE OVARIES, BUT DRAW THE EGG INTO THE TUBE BY MEANS OF FRINGES CALLED FIMBRIAE.

AT BIRTH, A HUMAN FEMALE HAS MORE THAN 400,000 IMMATURE OÖCYTES. OVER HER LIFETIME, ONLY AROUND 400 TO 450 WILL EVER BE RELEASED.

THE FEMALE CYCLE

LET'S BEGIN WITH THE BRAIN. IT SENDS A CHEMICAL SIGNAL TO THE OVARIES THAT CAUSES 10-20 OVARIAN FOLLICLES TO SWELL UP.

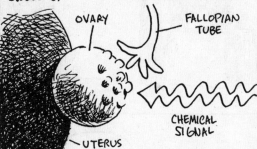

OVARY
FALLOPIAN TUBE
CHEMICAL SIGNAL
UTERUS

THE SWELLING FOLLICLES SECRETE A HORMONE CALLED ESTROGEN THAT CAUSES THE UTERINE WALL (ENDOMETRIUM) TO THICKEN WITH BLOOD-RICH TISSUE.

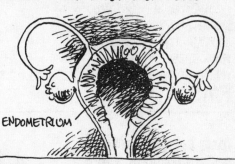

ENDOMETRIUM

AFTER ABOUT 9 DAYS, AN OVARIAN FOLLICLE POPS OUT AN OÖCYTE (UNFERTILIZED EGG), WHICH IS SWEPT INTO THE FALLOPIAN TUBE BY THE FIMBRIAE. THE OTHER FOLLICLES CONTINUE TO SECRETE ESTROGEN.

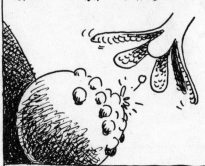

IF A SPERM ARRIVES AND CONCEPTION OCCURS, THE FERTILIZED EGG DROPS INTO THE UTERUS, WHERE A WARM, NOURISHING ENVIRONMENT IS MAINTAINED BY ANOTHER HORMONE, PROGESTERONE, RELEASED BY THE RUPTURED FOLLICLE.

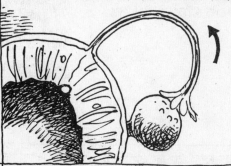

IF PREGNANCY DOES NOT OCCUR, HORMONE LEVELS DROP, AND THE THICKENED UTERINE LINING BEGINS TO BREAK UP.

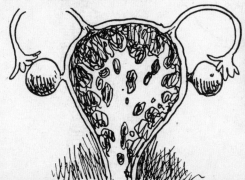

FINALLY, THE UTERUS FLUSHES THE EGG, ALONG WITH BLOOD, MUCUS, AND OTHER SECRETIONS — THE **MENSES** — WHICH FLOW OUT THE VAGINA.

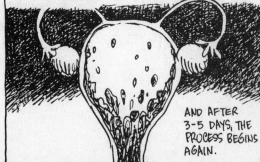

AND AFTER 3-5 DAYS, THE PROCESS BEGINS AGAIN.

43

THOSE 3-5 DAYS OF OUTFLOW — THE MENSTRUAL PERIOD — ARE A REGULAR EVENT IN THE LIVES OF MOST WOMEN. THEY MAY FEEL PHYSICAL DISCOMFORT: CRAMPS, BLOATING, TENDER BREASTS... OR HORMONE-INDUCED MOOD SWINGS, DEPRESSION, IRRITABILITY... IN EXTREME FORM THESE ARE CALLED PREMENSTRUAL SYNDROME, OR **PMS.**

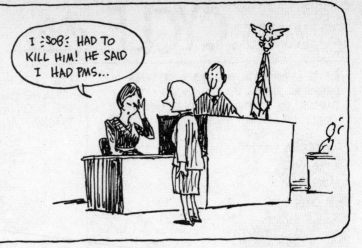

MOST CULTURES SURROUND MENSTRUATION WITH SOME TABOO, SINCE IT'S SO MYSTERIOUS, MOON-LINKED, AND BLOODY. SOME VIEW MENSTRUATING WOMEN AS HAVING SPECIAL POWERS.

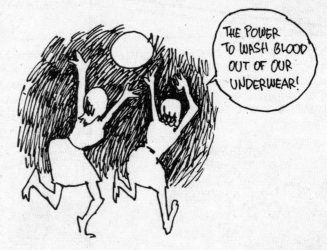

THIS FEAR OF MENSTRUATION CAN BECOME A FEAR OF THE VAGINA ITSELF. ALL OVER THE WORLD, THERE IS A MALE FANTASY THAT VAGINAS CONTAIN SOMETHING DANGEROUS, LIKE TEETH, OR WORSE.

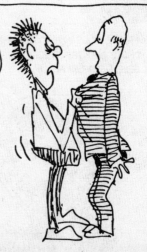

44

ANOTHER ORGAN, SEXY IF NOT EXACTLY SEXUAL, IS THE BREAST. THE FEMALE BREAST TAKES PART IN REPRODUCTION, SINCE IT NOURISHES OFFSPRING BY MAKING MILK. WITHIN THE BREAST, FATTY TISSUE CUSHIONS 15-20 MILK GLANDS WITH DUCTS LEADING TO THE NIPPLE.

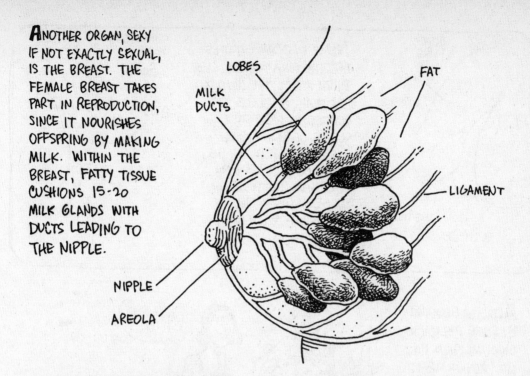

LOBES

MILK DUCTS

FAT

LIGAMENT

NIPPLE

AREOLA

THE BREAST IS HIGHLY SENSITIVE, ESPECIALLY THE NIPPLE, WHICH MAY BECOME ERECT IN RESPONSE TO COLD, TOUCH, OR SEXUAL AROUSAL. SOME MOTHERS REPORT THAT NURSING CAN BE QUITE EROTIC, WHICH IS WHY WE DON'T ALLOW 12 YEAR OLDS TO BREAST FEED.

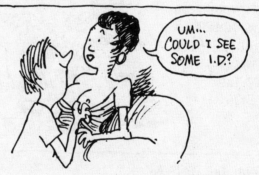

UM... COULD I SEE SOME I.D.?

OUR SOCIETY IS ALL MIXED UP ABOUT BREASTS—ARE THEY SEXY OR NURTURING? WELL, BOTH, AND SO NURSING IN PUBLIC IS ILLEGAL IN SOME STATES.

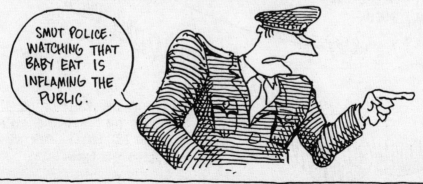

SMUT POLICE. WATCHING THAT BABY EAT IS INFLAMING THE PUBLIC.

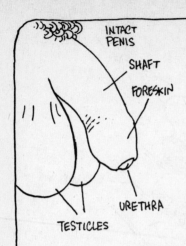

INTACT PENIS

SHAFT

FORESKIN

URETHRA

TESTICLES

MALE EXTERNAL GENITALS ARE THE PENIS AND TESTICLES. WHEN INTACT, THE HEAD OF THE PENIS, OR GLANS, IS COVERED BY A SENSITIVE SLEEVE OF SKIN CALLED THE FORESKIN. IN THE U.S., ABOUT 60% OF NEWBORN BOYS HAVE THE FORESKIN SURGICALLY REMOVED, BY AN OPERATION CALLED CIRCUMCISION.

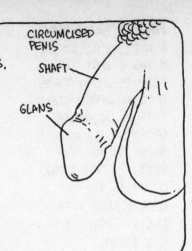

CIRCUMCISED PENIS

SHAFT

GLANS

ALTHOUGH REQUIRED BY SOME RELIGIONS, CIRCUMCISION HAS NO PROVEN HEALTH BENEFITS THAT CAN NOT BE ACHIEVED BY SIMPLE HYGIENE, I.E., WASHING UNDER THE FORESKIN.

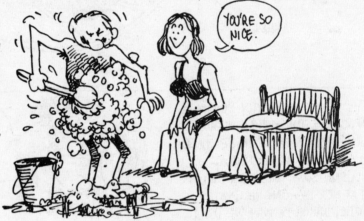

YOU'RE SO NICE.

WITHIN THE PENIS ARE THREE COLUMNS OF SPONGY TISSUE THAT FILL WITH BLOOD DURING SEXUAL AROUSAL, CAUSING ERECTION.

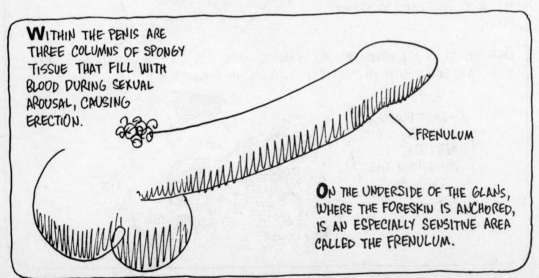

FRENULUM

ON THE UNDERSIDE OF THE GLANS, WHERE THE FORESKIN IS ANCHORED, IS AN ESPECIALLY SENSITIVE AREA CALLED THE FRENULUM.

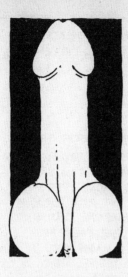

IN WORLD ART, OUTRAGEOUS PENISES OFTEN APPEAR AS SYMBOLS OF FERTILITY AND POWER. CONVERSELY, IMPOTENCE — LACK OF POWER — ALSO MEANS AN INABILITY TO GET AN ERECTION. THE MOST EXTREME FORM IS KORO, A DISEASE IN WHICH A MAN BELIEVES HIS PENIS IS SHRINKING TO NOTHINGNESS. (KORO HAS NO PHYSICAL BASIS.)

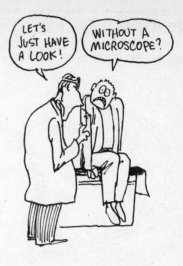

THIS BRINGS UP THE QUESTION: DOES SIZE MATTER? NO QUESTION HAS PROVOKED MORE MALE ANXIETY OVER THE AGES.

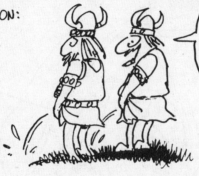

WELL, DOES IT?

HERE ARE SOME FACTS:

1) PENIS SIZE IS HEREDITARY.
2) IT IS NOT RELATED TO MASCULINITY OR SEXUAL ORIENTATION.
3) IT IS NOT RELATED TO NOSE LENGTH.
4) LIMP ONES VARY CONSIDERABLY IN LENGTH; ERECT ONES ARE MORE ALIKE.
5) PENIS SIZE DOES NOT AFFECT A MAN'S ABILITY TO HAVE INTERCOURSE OR PLEASE HIS PARTNER.
6) DESPITE #5, SOME WOMEN DO CARE!
7) DITTO FOR GAY MEN.
8) WHAT CAN YOU DO ABOUT IT, ANYWAY?

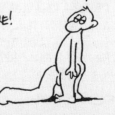

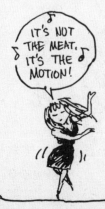

INTERNALLY, THE MALE REPRODUCTIVE ORGANS FORM A SPERM PRODUCTION AND DELIVERY SYSTEM. SPERM IS MADE IN THE TESTES AND TRAVELS THROUGH A LOOPING TUBE TO THE PENIS. ALONG THE WAY, A MIXTURE OF FLUIDS IS ADDED.

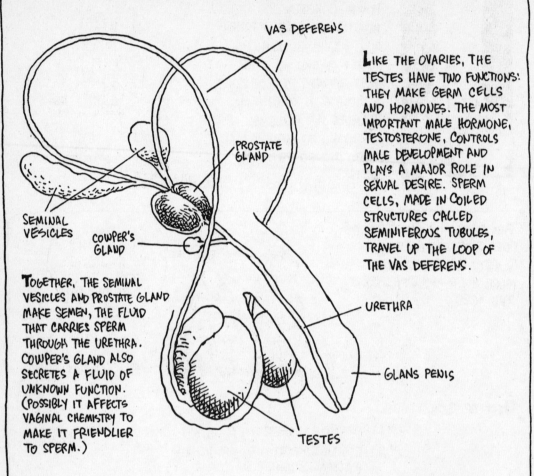

VAS DEFERENS

PROSTATE GLAND

SEMINAL VESICLES

COWPER'S GLAND

URETHRA

GLANS PENIS

TESTES

LIKE THE OVARIES, THE TESTES HAVE TWO FUNCTIONS: THEY MAKE GERM CELLS AND HORMONES. THE MOST IMPORTANT MALE HORMONE, TESTOSTERONE, CONTROLS MALE DEVELOPMENT AND PLAYS A MAJOR ROLE IN SEXUAL DESIRE. SPERM CELLS, MADE IN COILED STRUCTURES CALLED SEMINIFEROUS TUBULES, TRAVEL UP THE LOOP OF THE VAS DEFERENS.

TOGETHER, THE SEMINAL VESICLES AND PROSTATE GLAND MAKE SEMEN, THE FLUID THAT CARRIES SPERM THROUGH THE URETHRA. COWPER'S GLAND ALSO SECRETES A FLUID OF UNKNOWN FUNCTION. (POSSIBLY IT AFFECTS VAGINAL CHEMISTRY TO MAKE IT FRIENDLIER TO SPERM.)

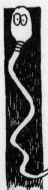

UNLIKE OVULATION, SPERMATOGENESIS (SPERM PRODUCTION) GOES ON ALL THE TIME. SPERM TAKE MORE THAN 70 DAYS TO DEVELOP, SHED MOST OF THEIR CELLULAR MASS, GROW A WHIPLIKE TAIL, AND MEANDER SLOWLY THROUGH THE EPIDIDYMIS BEFORE FINALLY REACHING THE VAS DEFERENS.

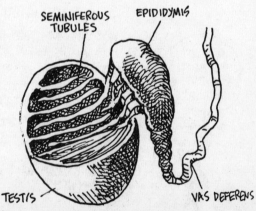

SEMINIFEROUS TUBULES

EPIDIDYMIS

TESTIS

VAS DEFERENS

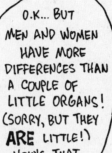

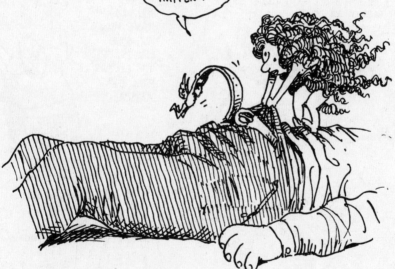

MORE ON HORMONES:

JUST LIKE WOMEN, MEN CAN BE EMOTIONALLY AFFECTED BY HORMONES. TESTOSTERONE TENDS TO MAKE MEN MORE AGGRESSIVE AND SELF-CONFIDENT.

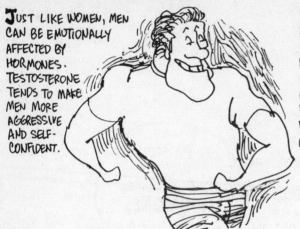

TESTOSTERONE RESPONDS TO CUES FROM THE ENVIRONMENT. IN THE FACE OF A CHALLENGE, FOR INSTANCE, IT TENDS TO GO UP.

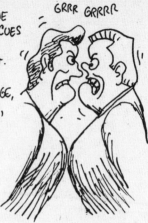

GRRR GRRRR

BEFORE A BIG GAME, ACCORDING TO ONE STUDY, PROFESSIONAL ATHLETES TEND TO HAVE VERY HIGH TESTOSTERONE LEVELS.

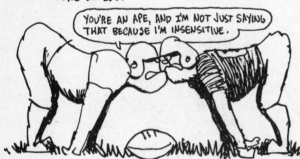

YOU'RE AN APE, AND I'M NOT JUST SAYING THAT BECAUSE I'M INSENSITIVE.

AFTER THE GAME, THE WINNERS (AND THEIR FANS!) STILL HAVE HIGH HORMONE LEVELS, BUT THE LOSERS' FALL DRAMATICALLY.

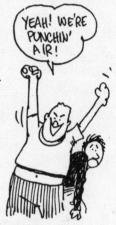

YEAH! WE'RE PUNCHIN' AIR!

TESTOSTERONE LEVELS FALL WITH DEFEAT, EXHAUSTION, SUBORDINATION, AND LACK OF CHALLENGE OR SEXUAL STIMULATION. SOLDIERS IN BOOT CAMP HAVE DEPRESSED LEVELS OF THE MALE HORMONE...

AND SO DO SETTLED, MONOGAMOUS MEN.

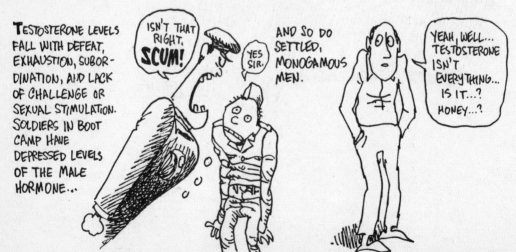

ISN'T THAT RIGHT, SCUM!

YES SIR.

YEAH, WELL... TESTOSTERONE ISN'T EVERYTHING... IS IT...? HONEY...?

50

HEIGHTENED TESTOSTERONE LEVELS ALSO GO WITH AN INTEREST IN SEX — IN BOTH FEMALES AND MALES. WOMEN MAKE TESTOSTERONE, BUT LESS OF IT. (BOTH "MALE" AND "FEMALE" HORMONES ARE MADE BY BOTH SEXES, BUT IN DIFFERENT AMOUNTS.)

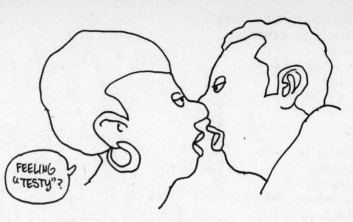

THESE HORMONES, WHICH SURGE DURING PUBERTY, TRIGGER DEVELOPMENTAL CHANGES: ESTROGEN PROMOTES BREAST GROWTH AND WIDENED HIPS, WHILE TESTOSTERONE CAUSES FACIAL HAIR, DEEPENING OF THE VOICE, AND EXTRA MUSCLE BULK. THESE EFFECTS VARY FROM ONE PERSON TO THE NEXT.

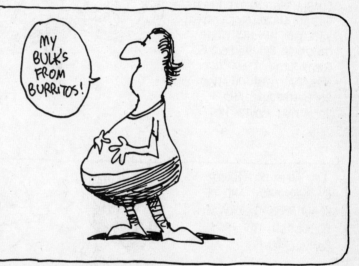

TAKING THE OTHER SEX'S HORMONES WILL CAUSE THE DEVELOPMENT OF THAT SEX'S CHARACTERISTICS. THIS IS ESPECIALLY HELPFUL IF YOU'RE A TRANSSEXUAL.

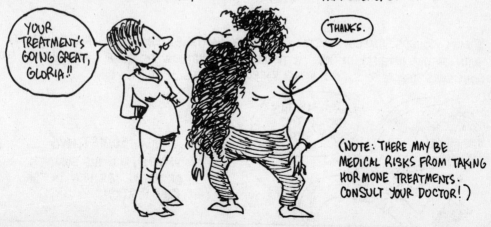

ALL RIGHT, THEN... THAT'S THE BASIC MACHINERY... NOW LET'S

TURN IT ON!

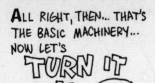

UM... WHERE'S THE SWITCH?

THE ON-OFF SWITCH, IT SEEMS, IS IN THE BRAIN!! DESIRE AND AROUSAL ORIGINATE IN THE LIMBIC SYSTEM, THE BRAIN'S EMOTIONAL CONTROL CENTER, WHICH IS HEAVILY WIRED TO OTHER BRAIN REGIONS CONTROLLING PERCEPTION, MEMORY, COMMUNICATION, UNDERSTANDING, AND VOLUNTARY MOVEMENT.

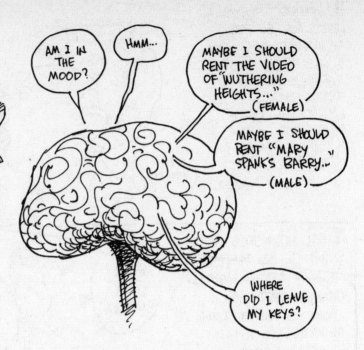

AM I IN THE MOOD?

HMM...

MAYBE I SHOULD RENT THE VIDEO OF "WUTHERING HEIGHTS..." (FEMALE)

MAYBE I SHOULD RENT "MARY SPANKS BARRY..." (MALE)

WHERE DID I LEAVE MY KEYS?

THE BRAIN IS AFFECTED BY HORMONES... AND THE BRAIN AFFECTS HORMONE PRODUCTION. IT'S VERY COMPLICATED!!

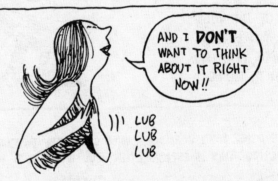

AND I **DON'T** WANT TO THINK ABOUT IT RIGHT NOW!!

LUB LUB LUB

SIGHTS, SOUNDS, SMELLS, TASTES, MEMORIES, FANTASIES, EMOTIONS — ALL COMBINE TO TURN ON OUR INTEREST IN SEX, OR TURN IT OFF. SOMETIMES THE SIGNALS ARE OBVIOUS, AND SOMETIMES THEY'RE SO SUBTLE WE'RE BARELY CONSCIOUS OF THEM.

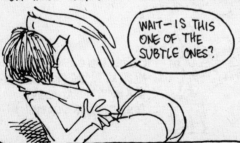

WAIT— IS THIS ONE OF THE SUBTLE ONES?

ANYWAY, **SOMETHING** HAPPENS, AND THE SWITCHES OF DESIRE ARE NOW IN THE **ON** POSITION.

IN BOTH MEN AND WOMEN, SEXUAL AROUSAL GOES THROUGH A STAGE OF INCREASING EXCITEMENT, WHICH CLIMAXES, IF WE'RE LUCKY, IN ORGASM.

GENERALLY, EXCITEMENT BRINGS SIMILAR PHYSICAL CHANGES TO BOTH SEXES: INCREASED BLOOD FLOW TO CERTAIN ORGANS (VASOCONGESTION) AND INVOLUNTARY MUSCLE TENSION (MYOTONIA). THE HEART RACES... THE FACE MAY FLUSH AND HEAT UP LIKE A STOVE...

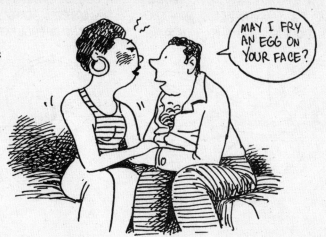

THOUGH THE PHYSICAL CHANGES ARE THE SAME FOR MOST PEOPLE, WHAT BRINGS THEM ON MAY DIFFER FROM ONE TO ANOTHER. IT MAY BE:

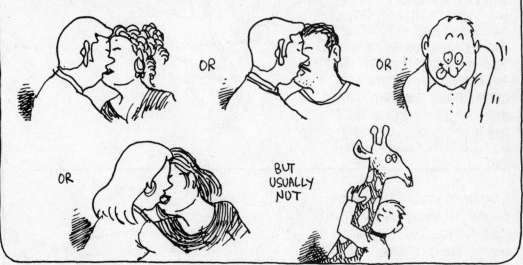

AND ONE OTHER THING: MEN USUALLY, BUT NOT ALWAYS, GET AROUSED FASTER THAN WOMEN.

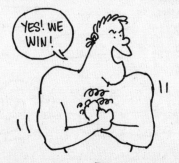

ON THE OTHER HAND, MALE STAYING POWER CAN LEAVE SOMETHING TO BE DESIRED. MORE ON THIS LATER...

MALES SHOW THE MOST DRAMATIC SIGN OF VASOCONGESTION: ERECTION. PENILE TISSUE FILLS WITH BLOOD, AND THE ORGAN DOUBLES OR TRIPLES IN SIZE.

AS EXCITEMENT PROGRESSES, THE TESTES RISE FURTHER, THE PROSTATE ENLARGES, AND COWPER'S GLAND SECRETES FLUID THAT MAY EMERGE AT THE TIP OF THE PENIS.

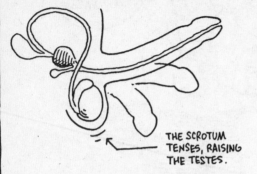

THE SCROTUM TENSES, RAISING THE TESTES.

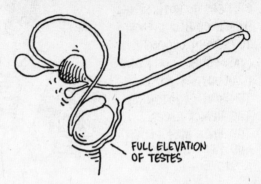

FULL ELEVATION OF TESTES

THEN, SUDDENLY, THE INTERNAL GLANDS BEGIN TO PULSE, PUMPING SEMEN TO THE URETHRA. THE MAN FEELS "EJACULATORY INEVITABILITY," THE SENSATION THAT GOING BACK IS IMPOSSIBLE. FINALLY, RAPID (EVERY 0.8 SECONDS) PULSING OF THE PROSTATE, URETHRA, AND MUSCLES AROUND THE BASE OF THE PENIS PUMP SEMEN AND SPERM OUT OF THE BODY IN SPURTS. THIS IS **EJACULATION**.

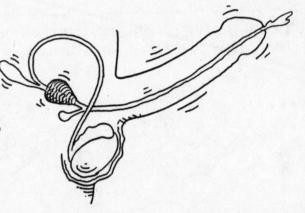

EJACULATION USUALLY GOES WITH ORGASM, AN INDESCRIBABLY INTENSE WAVE OF PLEASURABLE SENSATION AND RELEASE OF TENSION. FOR SOME TIME AFTER ORGASM, ERECTION AND ORGASM ARE IMPOSSIBLE. THIS SO-CALLED REFRACTORY PERIOD OR *PETIT MORT* ("LITTLE DEATH") CAN LAST FOR MINUTES, HOURS, OR EVEN DAYS IN OLDER MEN.

WHO'S COUNTING?

IN EARLY FEMALE AROUSAL, INTERNALLY THE VAGINA BEGINS SECRETING A CLEAR LUBRICATING FLUID, AND THE UTERUS BEGINS TO TIP UPWARD.

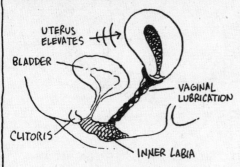

UTERUS ELEVATES

BLADDER

VAGINAL LUBRICATION

CLITORIS

INNER LABIA

AS STIMULATION CONTINUES, THE LOWER VAGINAL WALLS SWELL, WHILE THE UPPER VAGINA EXPANDS. THE UTERUS TIPS UP FURTHER.

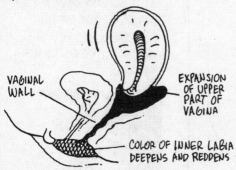

VAGINAL WALL

EXPANSION OF UPPER PART OF VAGINA

COLOR OF INNER LABIA DEEPENS AND REDDENS

AN ORGASM BRINGS RHYTHMIC CONTRACTIONS OF VAGINA, UTERUS, AND PELVIC MUSCLES ... AND BRINGS INTENSELY PLEASURABLE SENSATIONS AND RELIEF OF TENSION.

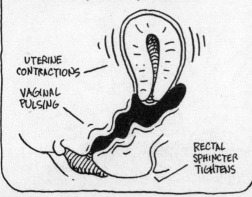

UTERINE CONTRACTIONS

VAGINAL PULSING

RECTAL SPHINCTER TIGHTENS

EXTERNALLY, AROUSAL'S VASOCONGESTION SWELLS THE CLITORIS AND THE LABIA MINORA. THE CLITORIS RETRACTS BENEATH ITS HOOD.

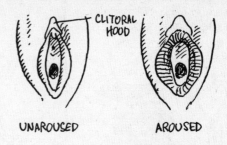

CLITORAL HOOD

UNAROUSED

AROUSED

AFTER ORGASM, THE CLITORIS REEMERGES, BUT IT REMAINS ENGORGED — ALLOWING MANY WOMEN (AROUND 15%) TO EXPERIENCE A SECOND ORGASM, OR EVEN MORE, RIGHT AWAY. THIS CAN BE A PROBLEM!

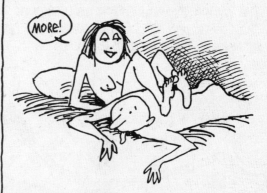

MORE!

ON THE OTHER HAND, SOME WOMEN HAVE TROUBLE REACHING ORGASM IN THE FIRST PLACE — ANOTHER POTENTIAL PROBLEM.

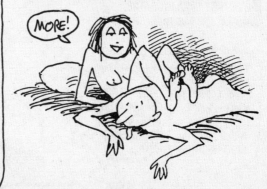

MORE!

THERE ARE MANY WAYS TO CAUSE AROUSAL AND ORGASM. THE REPRODUCTIVE WAY IS TO BRING PENIS AND VAGINA TOGETHER.

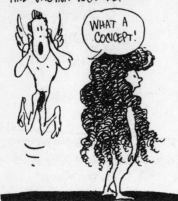

WHAT A CONCEPT!

SHAPE ASIDE, EACH ORGAN HAS FEATURES THAT WORK ON THE OTHER.

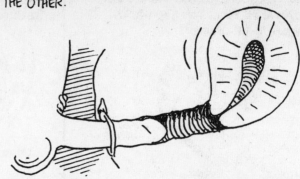

SEMEN CONTAINS CHEMICALS THAT BUFFER THE VAGINA (I.E. MAKE VAGINAL JUICES MORE SPERM-FRIENDLY) AND OTHER CHEMICALS, PROSTAGLANDINS, THAT PROMOTE VAGINAL AND UTERINE CONTRACTION — I.E., ORGASM.

THE VAGINA, MEANWHILE, SECRETES LUBRICANTS TO EASE THE PENIS'S WAY, SWELLS TO SQUEEZE THE PENIS, AND STRAIGHTENS THE PATH TO THE UTERUS.

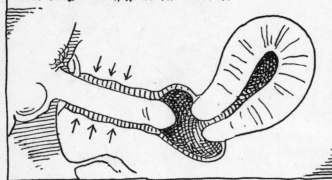

IT SOMETIMES HAPPENS THAT AFTER AN ACT OF THIS OLD-FASHIONED RITUAL, AN ERRANT SPERM LOCATES AN EGG...

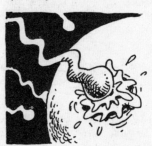

BUT THAT WOULD BE THE SUBJECT OF ANOTHER CHAPTER...

BY THE WAY, AREN'T YOU GLAD I DIDN'T MAKE PEOPLE DO IT LIKE THE BEES AND THE FLOWERS?

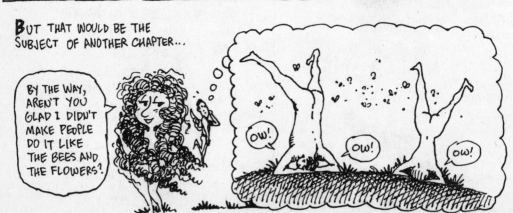

OW!

OW!

OW!

∘ CHAPTER 4 ∘
GROWING UP SEXUAL

LOOK! IT'S A
LITTLE BABY! ISN'T
IT CUTE? SO INNOCENT...
SO UNAWARE... AND
WHAT'S THE FIRST
QUESTION PEOPLE
WILL ASK ABOUT IT?
THE FIRST THING THEY
WANT TO KNOW?
SOMETHING ABOUT
SEX, NATURALLY...

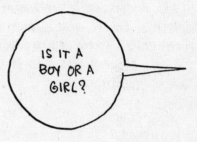

IS IT A
BOY OR A
GIRL?

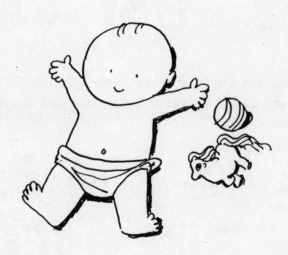

Is IT A BOY,
OR IS IT A
GIRL? THAT'S
THE FIRST
THING PEOPLE
WANT TO KNOW
ABOUT A
BABY.

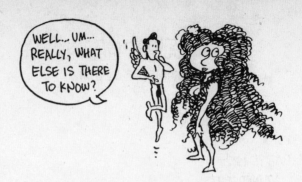

WELL... UM...
REALLY, WHAT
ELSE IS THERE
TO KNOW?

A FAMOUS PSYCHOLOGICAL EXPERIMENT SHOWED HOW BADLY WE WANT THE ANSWER.
A NUMBER OF ADULTS WERE DIVIDED INTO THREE GROUPS, AND EACH WAS SHOWN A
DIAPERED BABY (SO ITS GENITALS WERE INVISIBLE). GROUP 1 WAS TOLD THE BABY
WAS A BOY; GROUP 2 WAS TOLD IT WAS A GIRL; AND GROUP 3 WAS TOLD NOTHING
ONE WAY OR THE OTHER.

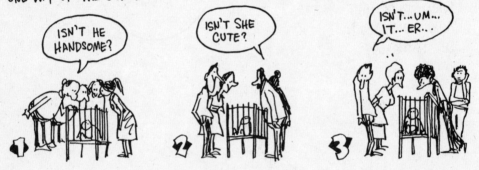

ISN'T HE
HANDSOME?

ISN'T SHE
CUTE?

ISN'T... UM...
IT... ER...

ASKED TO DESCRIBE THE BABIES' ACTIVITIES, THE GROUPS INTERPRETED THE SAME
BEHAVIOR IN DIFFERENT WAYS. FUSSINESS, FOR EXAMPLE, WAS CALLED "ANGER" BY GROUP 1
AND "FRUSTRATION" BY GROUP 2.

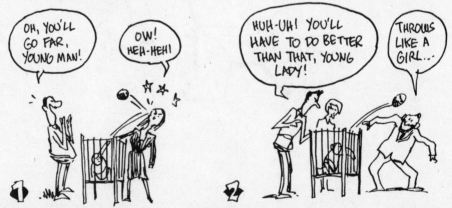

OH, YOU'LL
GO FAR,
YOUNG MAN!

OW!
HEH-HEH!

HUH-UH! YOU'LL
HAVE TO DO BETTER
THAN THAT, YOUNG
LADY!

THROWS
LIKE A
GIRL...

58

THE THIRD GROUP
SEEMED COMPLETELY
CONFUSED! THEY KEPT
TRYING TO FIGURE
OUT WHETHER THE
BABY WAS A BOY OR
A GIRL, BASED ON
HOW IT LOOKED
AND ACTED.

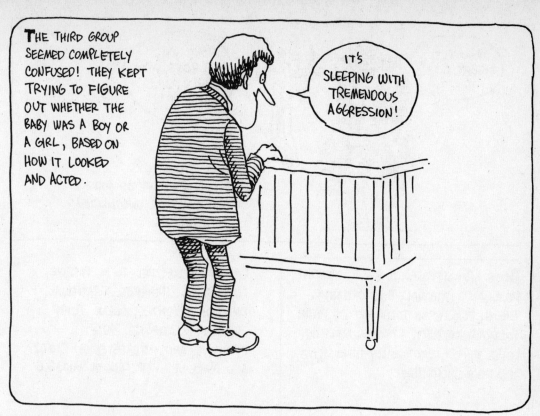

IT'S
SLEEPING WITH
TREMENDOUS
AGGRESSION!

THE PSYCHOLOGISTS CONCLUDED:
GROWN-UPS DESPERATELY
WANT TO KNOW THE BABY'S
SEX SO THEY CAN RELATE
TO THE CHILD "CORRECTLY."
THIS WAY, ADULTS HELP
TEACH THE BABY THE "RIGHT"
WAY TO BEHAVE. IF ADULTS
DON'T KNOW "WHAT IT IS,"
THEY GET VERY UNCOMFORTABLE!

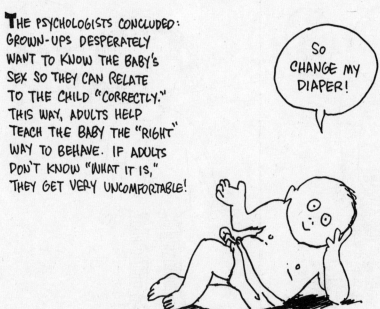

SO
CHANGE MY
DIAPER!

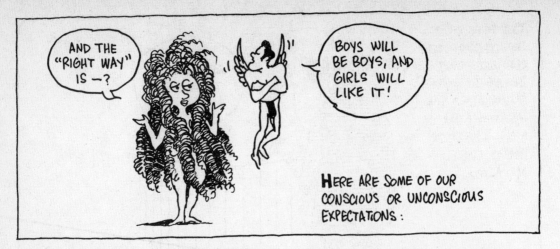

Here are some of our conscious or unconscious expectations:

Boys are supposed to be aggressive, dominant, rational, task-oriented, tough, fearless, tolerant of pain, tolerant of dirt, strong, athletic, loud, direct, emotionally insensitive, and have short hair.

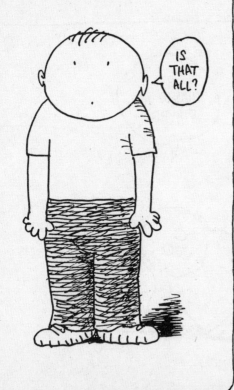

Girls are supposed to be passive, submissive, indirect, irrational, emotion-oriented, clean, soft, fearful, nurturing, quiet, intuitive, and interested in clothes and make-up. Hair length variable.

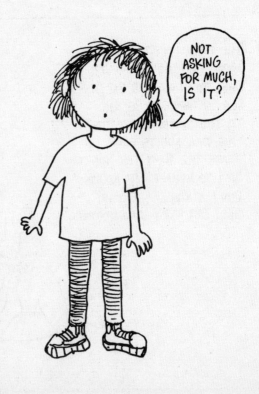

AND SO, BOYS HAVE TRADITIONALLY BEEN RAISED TO BE ROUGH AND TOUGH...

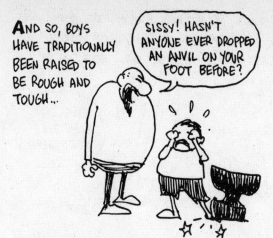

SISSY! HASN'T ANYONE EVER DROPPED AN ANVIL ON YOUR FOOT BEFORE?

WHILE GIRLS ARE TREATED MORE GENTLY.

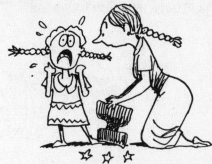

OH, HONEY, DO YOU HAVE AN OWIE?

BOYS GET "MASCULINE" TOYS, LIKE BLOCKS, TRUCKS, AND "ACTION FIGURES"... GIRLS GET TEA SETS AND DOLLS.

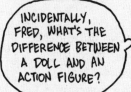

INCIDENTALLY, FRED, WHAT'S THE DIFFERENCE BETWEEN A DOLL AND AN ACTION FIGURE?

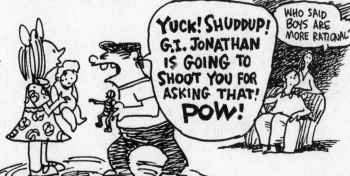

YUCK! SHUDDUP! G.I. JONATHAN IS GOING TO SHOOT YOU FOR ASKING THAT! POW!

WHO SAID BOYS ARE MORE RATIONAL?

IN THIS WAY, SOCIETY TEACHES EACH CHILD A **GENDER ROLE:** THE PART THE CHILD IS EXPECTED TO PLAY IN LIFE, DEPENDING ON WHICH SET OF GENITALS HAPPEN TO BE IN ITS POSSESSION.

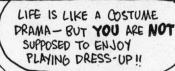

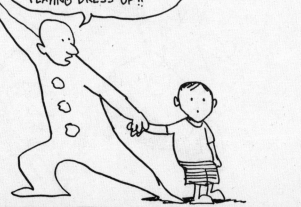

LIFE IS LIKE A COSTUME DRAMA — BUT **YOU** ARE **NOT** SUPPOSED TO ENJOY PLAYING DRESS-UP!!

BUT IN REALITY, BOYS AND GIRLS, MEN AND WOMEN, ARE NOT REALLY OPPOSITES, BUT SIMILAR IN MANY WAYS. MOST PEOPLE ARE A COMBINATION OF "MASCULINE" AND "FEMININE" QUALITIES. GIRLS CAN BE ASSERTIVE AND DECISIVE, WHILE BOYS CAN BE NURTURING AND COMPASSIONATE.

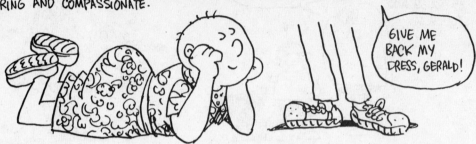

MODERN, HUMANISTIC-TYPE PARENTS RECOGNIZE THIS! THEY TRY TO TREAT CHILDREN EQUALLY AND GIVE THEM AN EQUAL CHANCE AT ALL THE TOYS.

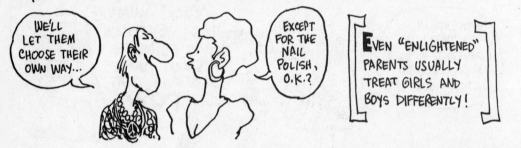

DESPITE THE FACT THAT PART OF OUR GENDER ROLE IS LEARNED, SOME OF IT SEEMS TO BE INNATE AS WELL. MANY A MODERN PARENT HAS BEEN DISMAYED TO SEE LITTLE JESSICA IGNORING HER TOY TRUCK IN FAVOR OF YOUNG JASON'S BARBIE DOLL, WHILE JASON CHASES THE FAMILY DOG WITH JESSICA'S HAMMER...

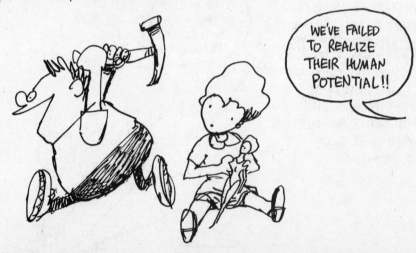

ANOTHER THING CHILDREN LEARN FROM INFANCY IS WHETHER BODIES ARE FOR TOUCHING.

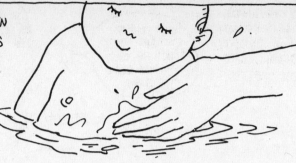

BABIES LOVE TO BE CUDDLED, TICKLED, AND STROKED, ESPECIALLY ON THEIR BARE SKIN, BUT WE USUALLY KEEP THEM DIAPERED, CLOTHED, BUNDLED...

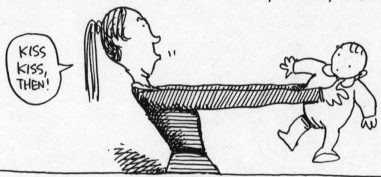

KISS KISS, THEN!

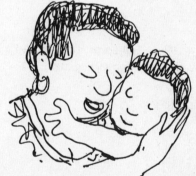

EITHER WAY, CHILDREN GENERALLY PICK UP THEIR PARENTS' ATTITUDE TOWARD SKIN-TO-SKIN CONTACT.

TOUCH-DEPRIVED CHILDREN GET USED TO DOING WITHOUT, BUT THEY TEND TO FEEL LESS SECURE THAN CUDDLED BABIES.

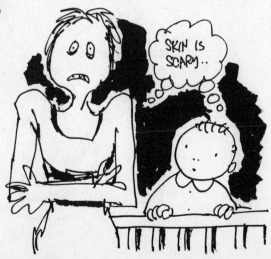

SKIN IS SCARY...

TOUCHING IS ONE THING...
SEX IS ANOTHER. SENSUALITY IS
DIFFERENT FROM SEXUALITY.
DO LITTLE CHILDREN HAVE
ACTUAL SEXUAL URGES?

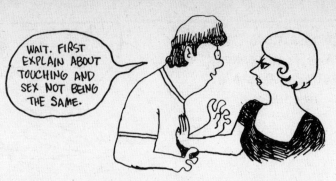

WAIT. FIRST
EXPLAIN ABOUT
TOUCHING AND
SEX NOT BEING
THE SAME.

IT'S AMAZING HOW MUCH DISAGREEMENT THIS QUESTION HAS PROVOKED... ONE TRADITIONAL
VIEW, FOR EXAMPLE, HOLDS THAT CHILDREN ARE VESSELS OF SIN, FULL OF IMPURITY AND
LUST, WHICH MOST BE CONTROLLED AND CORRECTED WITH THE UTMOST VIGILANCE.

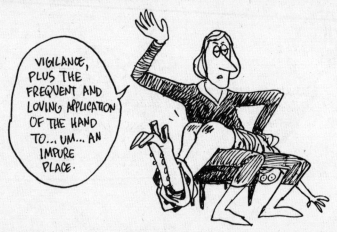

VIGILANCE,
PLUS THE
FREQUENT AND
LOVING APPLICATION
OF THE HAND
TO... UM... AN
IMPURE
PLACE.

ON THE OTHER HAND, IN VICTORIAN ENGLAND OF THE LATE 1800s, CHILDREN WERE THOUGHT
TO BE WHOLLY PURE AND INNOCENT. PROTECTING THEM FROM IMPURE SIGHTS AND
THOUGHTS WAS THE WAY TO GO!

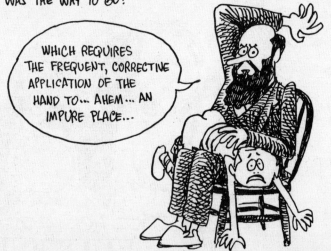

WHICH REQUIRES
THE FREQUENT, CORRECTIVE
APPLICATION OF THE
HAND TO... AHEM... AN
IMPURE PLACE...

VERY, VERY, VERY
DIFFERENT!!!

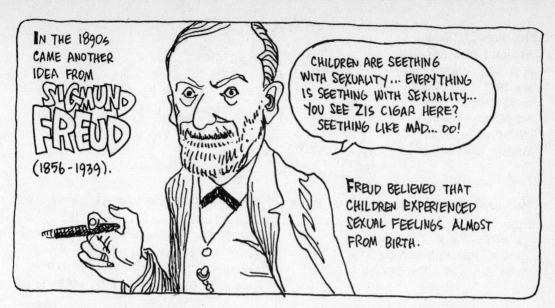

IN THE 1890s CAME ANOTHER IDEA FROM **SIGMUND FREUD** (1856-1939).

CHILDREN ARE SEETHING WITH SEXUALITY... EVERYTHING IS SEETHING WITH SEXUALITY... YOU SEE ZIS CIGAR HERE? SEETHING LIKE MAD... OO!

FREUD BELIEVED THAT CHILDREN EXPERIENCED SEXUAL FEELINGS ALMOST FROM BIRTH.

BUT UNLIKE THE OLD-TIME RELIGION, FREUD DID NOT BELIEVE IN BOTTLING THESE FEELINGS UP! AS A MATTER OF FACT, HE SAID THAT REPRESSION OF SEXUALITY WAS AT THE ROOT OF ALL NEUROSIS.

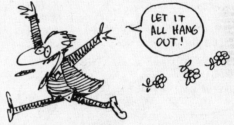

LET IT ALL HANG OUT!

MUCH OF FREUD'S THEORY HAS BEEN CHALLENGED, DEBUNKED, AND DISCARDED IN RECENT YEARS, SO WE WON'T GO INTO THE DETAILS...

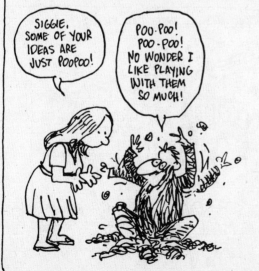

SIGGIE, SOME OF YOUR IDEAS ARE JUST POOPOO!

POO-POO! POO-POO! NO WONDER I LIKE PLAYING WITH THEM SO MUCH!

BUT THE FREUDIAN LEGACY LIVES ON IN TWO WIDELY-HELD IDEAS:

- **Children have sexuality.**
- **Repression is bad.**

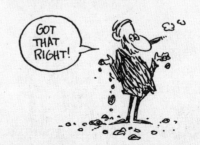

GOT THAT RIGHT!

How DOES CHILDHOOD SEXUALITY DEVELOP? WELL... MOST KIDS QUICKLY FIGURE OUT THAT IT FEELS GOOD "DOWN THERE." (AN ACCIDENT OF ANATOMY, BY THE WAY—MOST ANIMALS CAN'T REACH!)

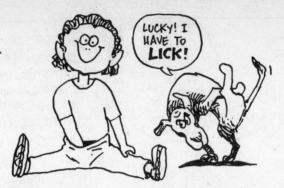

BUT WHAT ARE THEY SUPPOSED TO DO ABOUT IT? KIDS GET SEXUAL MESSAGES FROM MANY SOURCES

PARENTS: TRY AS THEY MIGHT, FEW PARENTS FEEL COMFORTABLE TALKING TO THEIR CHILDREN ABOUT SEX.

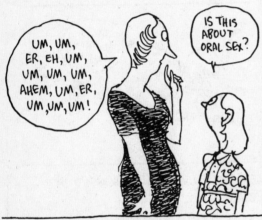

PROFESSIONAL SEX EDUCATORS: MOST OF THEM BELIEVE IN BEING OPEN ABOUT SEX (IN AN "AGE-APPROPRIATE" WAY). THIS MAY PUT THEM IN DIRECT CONFLICT WITH PARENTS.

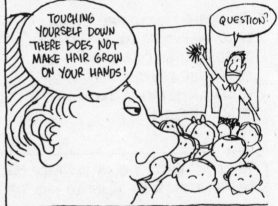

EACH OTHER: KIDS PLAY THE GAMES, SING THE SONGS, AND TELL THE JOKES THAT PASS DOWN THE LORE OF GENERATIONS PAST!

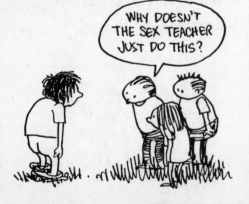

THE MEDIA: WHAT CAN WE SAY?

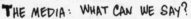

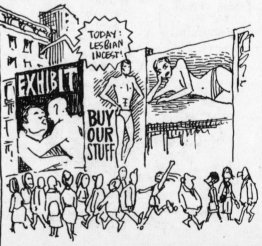

SINCE PEOPLE TAKE SO MANY
YEARS TO GROW UP, WE
HAVE WAY TOO MUCH TIME
TO TAKE IN ALL THOSE
MESSAGES AND IMAGES,
UNTIL OUR MINDS ARE
LOADED WITH SEXUAL
CONTRADICTIONS!

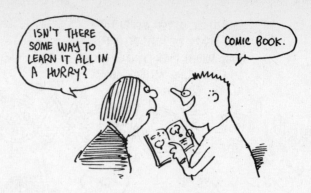

ISN'T THERE SOME WAY TO LEARN IT ALL IN A HURRY?

COMIC BOOK.

IF YOU BELIEVE EVERYTHING THAT'S THROWN AT US, ALL THIS MUST BE TRUE:

SEXUALITY IS NATURAL AND PLEASURABLE.

SEXUALITY IS SHAMEFUL AND EVIL.

SEX BEFORE MARRIAGE IS O.K.

SEX BEFORE MARRIAGE IS SINFUL.

SEX WITHIN MARRIAGE IS HOLY.

SEX WITHIN MARRIAGE IS RARE.

YOU SHOULD ALWAYS BE FULLY CLOTHED,
    EXCEPT DURING SEX.

EVERYTHING IS O.K. IN PUBLIC,
    EXCEPT SEX.

BOYS RULE.

GIRLS RULE.

BOYS AND GIRLS ARE EQUAL.

BLONDE GIRLS WITH LARGE BREASTS
    ARE ESPECIALLY EQUAL.

SEX IS FUN.

SEX IS RISKY.

THE IDEAL WOMAN IS:
    AN ANOREXIC MODEL
    A CURVY PLAYBOY CENTERFOLD
    ROSEANNE.

THE IDEAL MAN IS:
    BLOND AND WITHOUT LIPS
    BLACK, WITH CHISELED MUSCLES AND NO NECK
    DANNY DEVITO.

ATTRACTION TO THE SAME SEX IS NATURAL.

ATTRACTION TO THE SAME SEX IS SICK, WRONG,
    OR CRIMINAL.

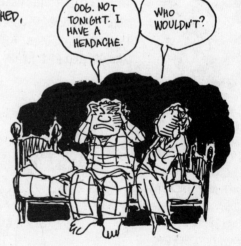

OOG. NOT TONIGHT. I HAVE A HEADACHE.

WHO WOULDN'T?

AND THEN, AFTER MORE THAN
TEN YEARS OF THIS STUFF,
JUST WHEN EVERYTHING LOOKS
AS CONFUSING AS POSSIBLE,
ALONG COME...

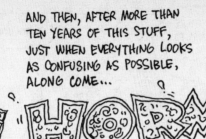

THE HORMONES!

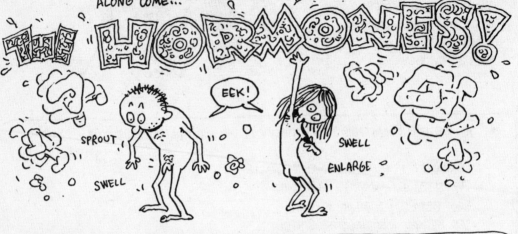

SPROUT

EEK!

SWELL

SWELL

ENLARGE

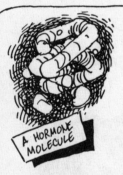

A HORMONE MOLECULE

SUDDENLY, OR FAIRLY SUDDENLY, THE BODY BEGINS CHURNING OUT THESE POTENT CHEMICALS — IN GIRLS, MAINLY ESTROGENS, IN BOYS MAINLY ANDROGENS, ESPECIALLY TESTOSTERONE — THE HORMONES TRIGGER CHANGES IN REPRODUCTIVE ORGANS, CAUSING THEM TO MATURE AND GET READY TO WORK...

IN BOYS, PENIS AND TESTICLES GROW... HEIGHT MAY INCREASE RAPIDLY... FEET AND HANDS GROW... THE VOICE DEEPENS... BODY HAIR SPROUTS...

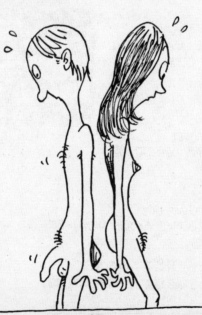

GIRLS ALSO HAVE A GROWTH SPURT... BREASTS DEVELOP... PUBIC AND UNDERARM HAIR APPEAR... AND VAGINAL SECRETIONS BEGIN.

THIS TRANSITION, KNOWN AS PUBERTY, BRINGS SOME BIG CHANGES:

BOYS, IF THEY HAVEN'T ALREADY, BEGIN TO HAVE ORGASMS WITH THE EJACULATION OF SEMEN.

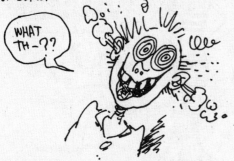

WHAT TH-??

BOTH SEXES, FOR SOME REASON, MAY DEVELOP SOME NEW BEHAVIORS, LIKE BLUSHING OR STAMMERING...

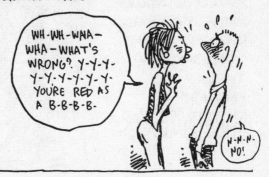

WH-WH-WHA-WHA-WHAT'S WRONG? Y-Y-Y-Y-Y-Y-Y-Y-Y YOU'RE RED AS A B-B-B-B-

N-N-N-NO!

AND EXCESSIVE GROOMING BEHAVIOR.

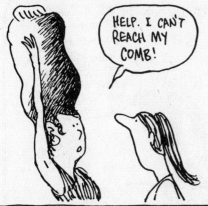

HELP. I CAN'T REACH MY COMB!

THEN THERE ARE THE PIMPLES.

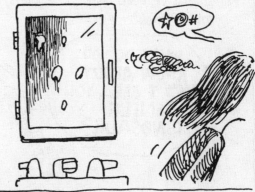

✜@#

GIRLS HAVE THEIR FIRST MENSTRUATION, OR MENARCHE. WHEN THIS HAPPENS (ANYTIME BETWEEN THE AGES OF 9 AND 17), IT IS A CLEAR SIGN OF IMPENDING WOMANHOOD. NOW A GIRL CAN BECOME PREGNANT.

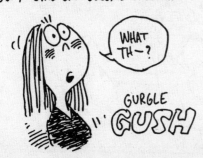

WHAT TH-?

GURGLE GUSH

UNFORTUNATELY, MANY EMBARRASSED MOMS "FORGET" TO TALK ABOUT IT AHEAD OF TIME, SO ABOUT 1/3 OF ADOLESCENT GIRLS DON'T KNOW WHAT'S HAPPENING WHEN THEY GET THEIR FIRST PERIOD.

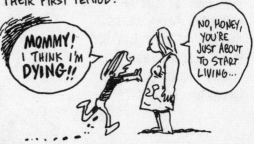

MOMMY! I THINK I'M DYING!!

NO, HONEY, YOU'RE JUST ABOUT TO START LIVING...

BEHOLD THE PUBERTAL
HUMAN... THE TEENAGER...
THE ADOLESCENT.
PHYSICALLY MATURE
(ALMOST), BUT NOT
MENTALLY OR SOCIALLY
MATURE. THEIR BODIES
SCREAM "DO IT!" BUT
SOCIETY SAYS "DON'T."
THE SENSE OF
FRUSTRATION IS
ENORMOUS!!

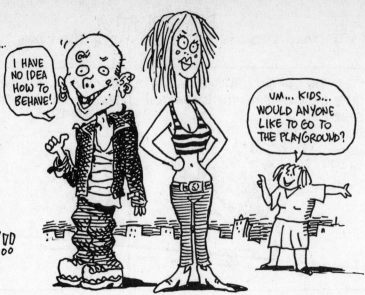

NO WONDER WE FEEL ANGRY, REBELLIOUS, AND CONTEMPTUOUS TOWARDS OUR PARENTS
AND OTHER AUTHORITY FIGURES!

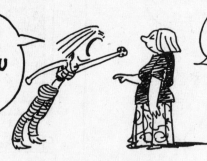

NOT TO MENTION THE ACUTE
SENSE OF DISAPPOINTMENT,
DESPAIR, AND SELF-LOATHING
THAT COME FROM COMPARING
OURSELVES TO BUFF AND
BEAUTIFUL MEDIA IDEALS...
THIS CAN BE ESPECIALLY BAD
IF WE ALREADY FEEL
INSECURE ABOUT OUR OWN
WORTH AND LOVABILITY.

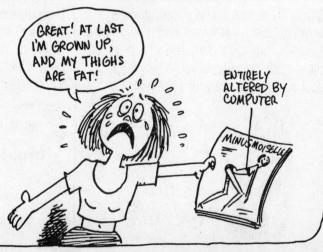

70

THE SENSE OF ISOLATION AND DESPAIR CAN BE ESPECIALLY ACUTE FOR GAY AND LESBIAN TEENS. THEY MAY BE TOO EMBARRASSED TO ADMIT THEIR SAME-SEX ATTRACTIONS TO ANYONE.

OH, WHY CAN'T I AFFORD A TICKET TO SAN FRANCISCO?

WHAT CAUSES OUR EROTIC FEELINGS TO BE DIRECTED TOWARD ONE SEX OR THE OTHER? NO ONE KNOWS FOR SURE... SOME PSYCHOLOGISTS, FOLLOWING FREUD, BELIEVE IT'S A MATTER OF UPBRINGING... OTHERS SUSPECT IT'S PROGRAMMED IN OUR GENES.

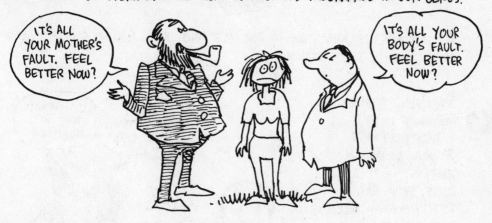

IT'S ALL YOUR MOTHER'S FAULT. FEEL BETTER NOW?

IT'S ALL YOUR BODY'S FAULT. FEEL BETTER NOW?

SINCE GAY TEENS, LIKE MOST TEENS, MOSTLY WANT TO FIT IN, THEY MAY FEEL AN EXTRA DOSE OF ANGST AROUND THIS QUESTION!

AM I NORMAL?

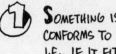
WHAT DOES "NORMAL" MEAN? AT LEAST TWO DIFFERENT THINGS...

1 **S**OMETHING IS NORMAL IF IT CONFORMS TO SOCIAL "NORMS," I.E., IF IT FITS IN WITH THE WAY SOCIETY SAYS THINGS **OUGHT** TO BE. FOR EXAMPLE, CHURCH, SYNAGOGUE, MOSQUE, AND THE GEORGIA LEGISLATURE HAVE ALL SAID AT ONE TIME OR ANOTHER THAT HOMOSEXUALITY IS WRONG AND ABNORMAL. "ABOMINATION" WAS ONE OF THEIR MILDER WORDS FOR IT.

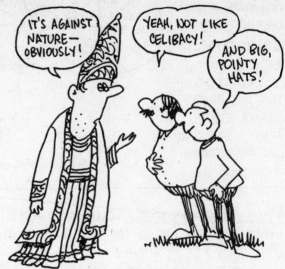

AS GAYS AND LESBIANS STRUGGLE FOR ACCEPTANCE, SOME RELIGIOUS DENOMINATIONS HAVE SOFTENED THEIR STANCE.

2 **S**OMETHING IS ALSO NORMAL IF IT FALLS WITHIN THE RANGE OF WHAT COMMONLY HAPPENS. IN THIS SENSE, BEING GAY IS TOTALLY NORMAL, BECAUSE HOMOSEXUALITY HAS ALWAYS EXISTED, EXISTS NOW, AND ALWAYS WILL EXIST.

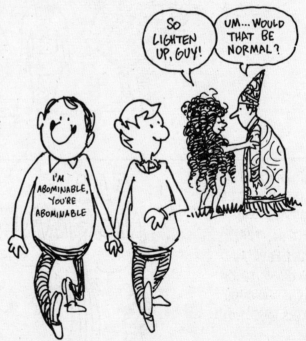

BESIDES COPING WITH CHANGING BODIES AND URGES, ADOLESCENTS ALSO HAVE TO LEARN HOW TO INTERACT SEXUALLY. SINCE WE ALMOST NEVER ACTUALLY SEE ANYONE DOING IT IN THE REAL WORLD, THIS CAN BE A BIT OF A CHALLENGE.

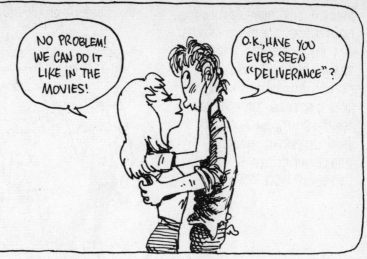

THE MOST COMMON SEXUAL ACTIVITY AMONG TEENAGERS HAS TO BE KISSING... THEN IT'S ON TO PETTING... AND, FOR SOME, INTERCOURSE. (ORAL SEX IS ALSO ON THE RISE AMONG TEENS, SINCE IT CAN'T CAUSE PREGNANCY.)

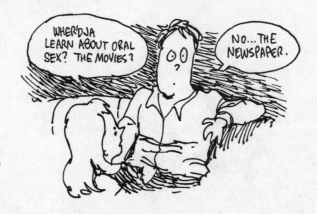

BUT SINCE TEENS ARE JUST BEGINNING TO FEEL THEIR WAY AROUND (SO TO SPEAK) AND DON'T HAVE WELL-DEVELOPED SEXUAL HABITS, THEY'RE NOT VERY GOOD AT USING BIRTH CONTROL OR PRACTICING SAFE SEX.

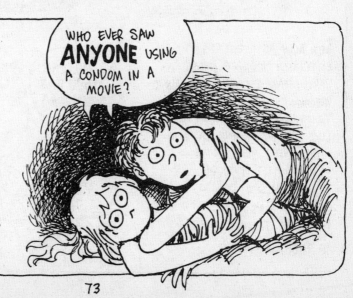

73

So... ON THE THRESHOLD OF
ADULTHOOD, THEIR IDENTITIES
NOT FULLY FORMED, WHAT DO
TEENAGERS DO? THEY
EXPERIMENT WITH DIFFERENT
ROLES, SETTING THEMSELVES
APART FROM MOM AND DAD
WITH DIFFERENT HAIR,
DIFFERENT CLOTHES, AND
DIFFERENT ACCESSORIES.

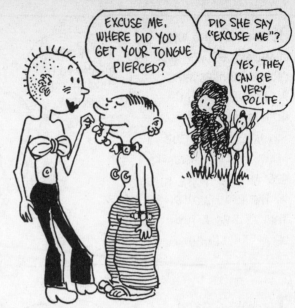

AND THEY TAKE **RISKS**ooo.... BY AGE 16, ABOUT HALF OF ALL TEENAGERS
HAVE ENGAGED IN SEX OF SOME KIND.

SOMETIMES IT'S A
RESULT OF PEER
PRESSURE...

AND SOMETIMES
IT'S PRESSURE
FROM OLDER
MEN...

SEXUALLY ACTIVE TEENS,
ESPECIALLY YOUNGER ONES,
RARELY TAKE PRECAUTIONS AGAINST
PREGNANCY OR SEXUALLY
TRANSMISSIBLE DISEASES (STDs)
LIKE HERPES, GONORRHEA, AND
AIDS. EVERY YEAR, SOME
3 MILLION NEW
CASES OF STDs — ABOUT
$\frac{1}{4}$ OF THE TOTAL — OCCUR
IN TEENAGERS.

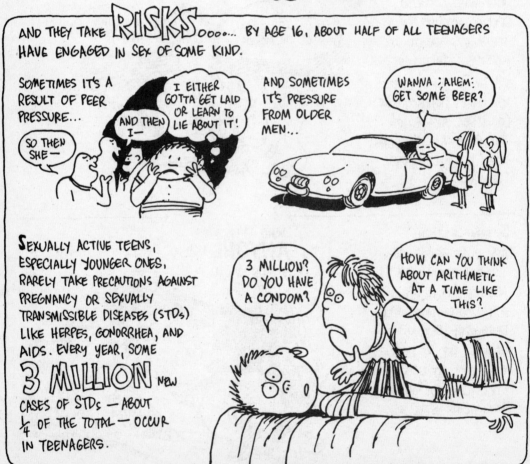

TEENS TAKE RISKS FOR SEVERAL REASONS:

THEY THINK THEY'RE INVULNERABLE AND DON'T WORRY ABOUT CONSEQUENCES.

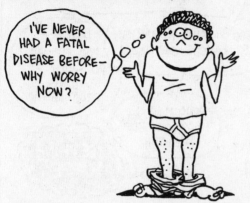

I'VE NEVER HAD A FATAL DISEASE BEFORE— WHY WORRY NOW?

SOMETIMES THEY'RE RAISED WITH POOR COMMUNICATION SKILLS...

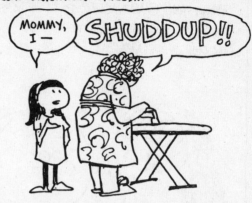

MOMMY, I —

SHUDDUP!!

...SO THAT WHEN IT COMES TIME TO TALK ABOUT SEXUAL ISSUES, THEY JUST CAN'T.

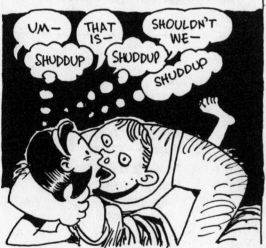

UM— THAT IS— SHOULDN'T WE—
SHUDDUP   SHUDDUP
SHUDDUP

AND SOMETIMES THEY'RE MORE ASHAMED OF TALKING ABOUT SEX THAN THEY ARE ABOUT DOING IT.

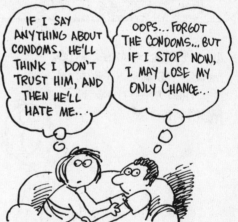

IF I SAY ANYTHING ABOUT CONDOMS, HE'LL THINK I DON'T TRUST HIM, AND THEN HE'LL HATE ME...

OOPS... FORGOT THE CONDOMS... BUT IF I STOP NOW, I MAY LOSE MY ONLY CHANCE...

THE GOOD NEWS IS THAT CONDOM USE AMONG TEENS IS RISING... THE BAD NEWS IS THAT RISK-TAKING AMONG SEXUALLY ACTIVE TEENS REMAINS THE NORM — IN SENSE #2.

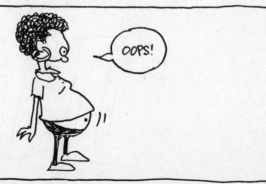

OOPS!

75

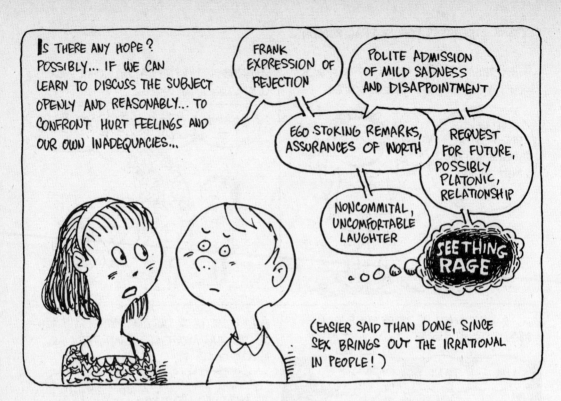

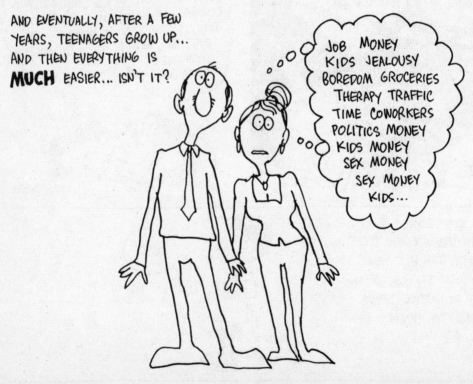

· CHAPTER 5 ·

WHO VACUUMS? GENDER AND SEXUALITY IN ADULT LIFE

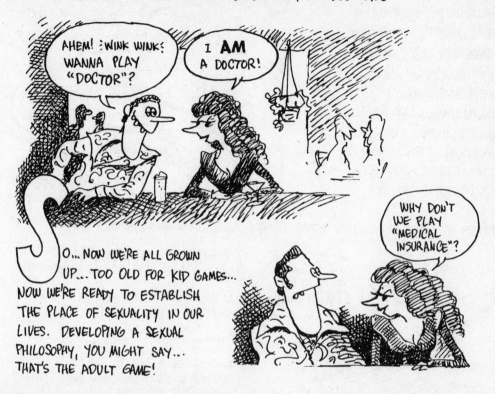

S...NOW WE'RE ALL GROWN UP...TOO OLD FOR KID GAMES... NOW WE'RE READY TO ESTABLISH THE PLACE OF SEXUALITY IN OUR LIVES. DEVELOPING A SEXUAL PHILOSOPHY, YOU MIGHT SAY... THAT'S THE ADULT GAME!

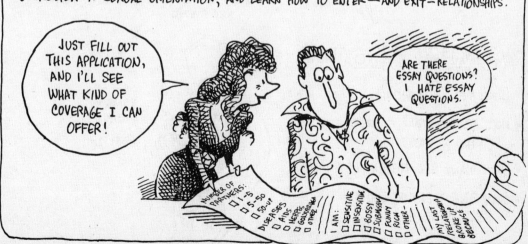

NOW WE MAKE CHOICES: WHEN TO DO IT, WHERE TO DO IT, HOW TO DO IT, WITH WHOM TO DO IT — OR EVEN WHETHER TO DO IT AT ALL. WE GRAPPLE WITH GENDER ROLES, ESTABLISH A SEXUAL ORIENTATION, AND LEARN HOW TO ENTER — AND EXIT — RELATIONSHIPS.

GENDER AND SEX

Growing up, we pick up ideas about traditional gender roles... we learn that masculine means aggressive, dominant, unemotional, and horny, while feminine means emotional, passive, and coy. How do these roles play out in the bedroom?

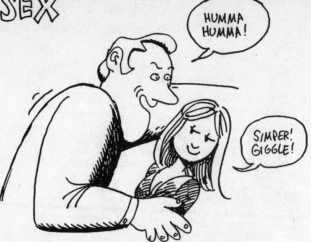

When it comes to sex, traditional gender roles go something like this:

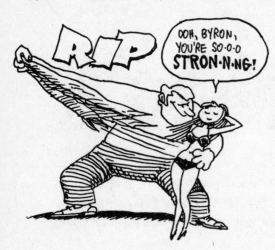

MEN SHOULD:

- ALWAYS LUST AFTER WOMEN, NEVER AFTER OTHER MEN.
- ALWAYS BE IN CHARGE.
- ALWAYS BE READY TO PERFORM LIKE A STALLION (AND BE EQUIPPED LIKE ONE).
- NEVER FEEL OR EXPRESS DOUBT OR REGRET.
- HAVE AN INNATE ABILITY TO UNHOOK BRA STRAPS.

WOMEN SHOULD:

- LIKE MEN, NOT WOMEN.
- NOT BE TOO OBVIOUS ABOUT LIKING A MAN.
- ONLY WANT SEX WITHIN MARRIAGE.
- ONLY GIVE PLEASURE, NOT RECEIVE IT.

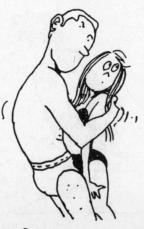

WOMEN SHOULD ALSO (THE FEMALE LIST IS LONGER!):

* NOT TOUCH THEMSELVES "DOWN THERE."

* ACHIEVE ORGASM AS A RESULT OF PENILE THRUSTING FROM ABOVE.

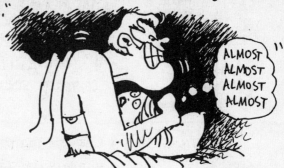

AND ALSO:

* LIE IF NECESSARY TO PROP UP THE FRAGILE MALE EGO.

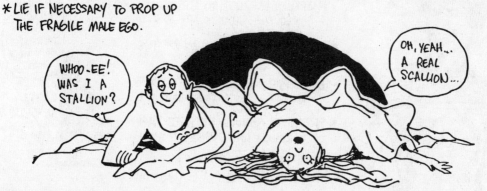

WELL... THIS TRADITIONAL SEXUAL ENCOUNTER CERTAINLY IS MALE-CENTERED! HE TAKES THE INITIATIVE, RUNS THE SHOW, AND QUITS WHEN HE WANTS... AND SO HE MAY CREATE MANY OPPORTUNITIES FOR FRUSTRATION, ANXIETY, ANGER, LINGERING RESENTMENT, AND MIS- OR NONCOMMUNICATION!

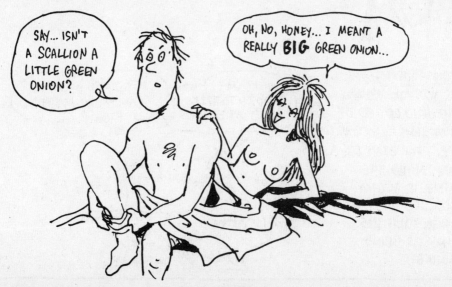

79

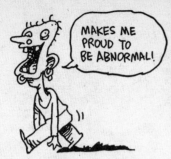

MAKES ME PROUD TO BE ABNORMAL!

So... ENOUGH IS ENOUGH... SINCE THE 1970s, WHEN THE WOMEN'S MOVEMENT CHALLENGED MALE SUPREMACY, WE HAVE MOVED INTO AN ERA OF MORE EQUAL AND **RELATIONSHIP-** CENTERED SEXUAL IDEAS. FOR EXAMPLE:

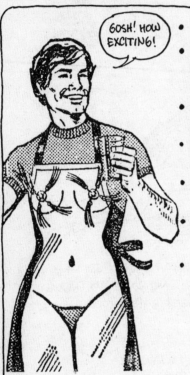

GOSH! HOW EXCITING!

- SAME-SEX PARTNERS ARE O.K.
- MUTUALLY AGREEABLE FORMS OF SEXUAL EXPRESSION BETWEEN (AMONG?) CONSULTING ADULTS ARE O.K.
- EITHER PARTNER CAN MAKE THE FIRST MOVE.
- BOTH PARTNERS ARE ENTITLED TO AN ORGASM, IF THEY WANT IT!
- PARTNERS SHOULD EXPRESS THEIR FEELINGS AND DESIRES OPENLY.
- PREMARITAL SEX IS O.K., AT LEAST WITHIN A RELATIONSHIP.
- CASUAL SEX ISN'T NECESSARILY BAD, BUT PROPER PRECAUTIONS AGAINST PREGNANCY AND DISEASE **MUST** BE TAKEN.

"AMONG"?

YES, YOU KNOW, IN CASE THERE ARE MORE THAN TWO.

FOR THESE IDEAS TO WORK, MEN AND WOMEN WILL HAVE TO LET GO OF SOME OF THEIR TRADITIONAL "STUFF." FOR EXAMPLE, A WOMAN TAKING THE INITIATIVE IS ACTING "MASCULINE," WHILE A MAN DISCUSSING HIS FEELINGS IS BEING "FEMININE."

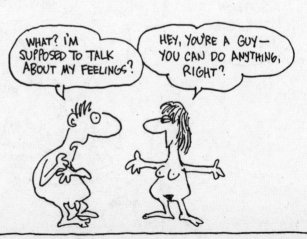

WHAT? I'M SUPPOSED TO TALK ABOUT MY FEELINGS?

HEY, YOU'RE A GUY— YOU CAN DO ANYTHING, RIGHT?

MIXING UP MASCULINE AND FEMININE TRAITS IN THIS WAY IS CALLED

ANDROGYNY

(FROM GREEK *ANDROS* = MAN, *GYNE* = WOMAN).

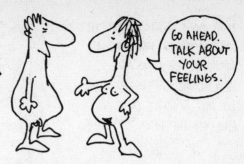

Go AHEAD. TALK ABOUT YOUR FEELINGS.

O.K...UM... I FEEL A LITTLE **WARM**... I FEEL LIKE WATCHING THE GAME ON **T.V.**...

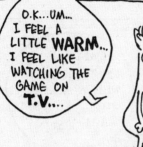

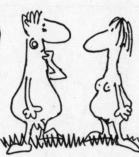

IN THE HEAT OF THE MOMENT AND THE HEIGHT OF THE MOVEMENT, SOME GENDER THEORISTS WENT SO FAR AS TO ADVOCATE **COMPLETE ANDROGYNY** AS THE KEY TO SEXUAL EQUALITY. IF EVERYONE ACTED ALIKE, THEY SAID, HOW COULD THERE BE A WAR BETWEEN THE SEXES?

LATER, MOST OF THESE FOLKS BACKED OFF THIS OPINION. AS ONE THEORIST PUT IT, IT WAS **TWICE** AS HARD TO BE PERFECTLY MALE **AND** FEMALE AS TO BE ONE OR THE OTHER!

I FEEL A PIMPLE ON MY CHIN... WOW! THIS TALKING ABOUT YOUR FEELINGS ISN'T SO HARD!

SMAK

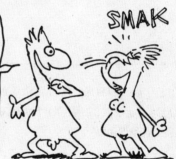

BY THE WAY, THE WAY YOU SMACKED YOUR FOREHEAD JUST NOW WAS VERY MASCULINE!

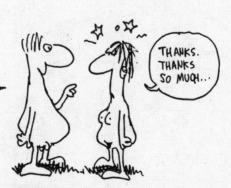

THANKS. THANKS SO MUCH...

For most people, complete androgyny is impossible, anyway. As long as hormonal differences exist, so will some of our gender differences.

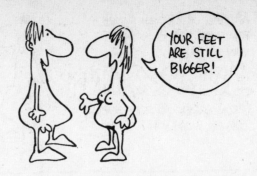

Besides, you have to wonder, if everyone had blended genders, would we still turn each other on as much as we do now?

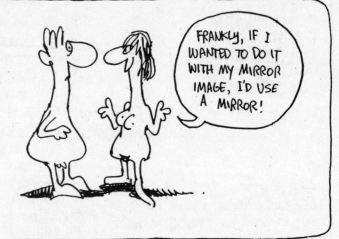

Still... a measure of androgyny can help open up lines of communication... reduce the pressure to play out the old roles... and maybe even spice up a relationship!!

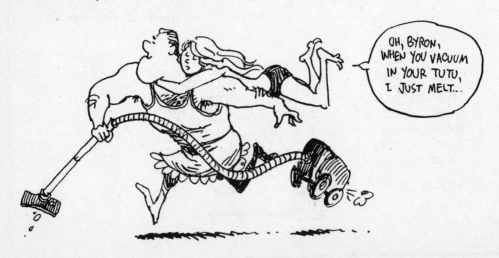

AND LET'S NOT FORGET THAT SOME PEOPLE REALLY ARE ANDROGYNOUS BIOLOGICALLY! AS WE SAW IN CHAPTER 3, A FEW BABIES ARE BORN WITH TWO SETS OF GENITALS OR AMBIGUOUS GENITALS.

FOR INSTANCE, THEY MAY BE FEMINIZED MALES: GENETICALLY MALE, BUT WITH SUCH LOW TESTOSTERONE LEVELS THAT THEY ALSO DEVELOP SOME FEMALE CHARACTERISTICS. AS WE SAW, DOCTORS HAVE BEEN QUICK TO CARVE THE PARTS TO MAKE THEM LOOK ENTIRELY FEMALE.

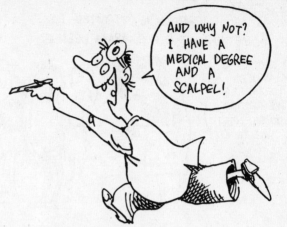

AND WHY NOT? I HAVE A MEDICAL DEGREE AND A SCALPEL!

THE PROBLEM IS SOME OF THESE PEOPLE MAY GROW UP FEELING LIKE BOYS!

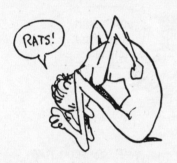

RATS!

THIS SENSATION OF FEELING LIKE ONE SEX TRAPPED IN THE BODY OF THE OTHER SEX GOES BY THE SCIENTIFIC NAME OF

GENDER DYSPHORIA.

NOT ALL GENDER DYSPHORICS ARE HORMONAL ANDROGYNES OR HERMAPHRODITES. SOME PEOPLE, FOR REASONS THAT ARE ARE HARD TO EXPLAIN, SIMPLY THINK OF THEMSELVES AS BELONGING TO THE OTHER SEX.

FOR THEM, A SEX CHANGE OPERATION MAY BE AN OPTION. AN ESTIMATED 70,000 PEOPLE WORLDWIDE HAVE HAD THEIR GENDER SURGICALLY SWITCHED. **warning**: DO NOT DO THIS WITHOUT EXTENSIVE COUNSELING!!!

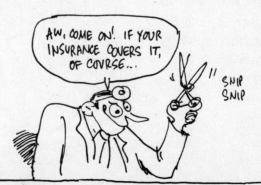

AW, COME ON! IF YOUR INSURANCE COVERS IT, OF COURSE...

SNIP SNIP

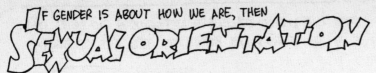

IF GENDER IS ABOUT HOW WE ARE, THEN **SEXUAL ORIENTATION** IS ABOUT WHAT WE'RE ATTRACTED TO... SOMETHING LIKE A COMPASS NEEDLE.

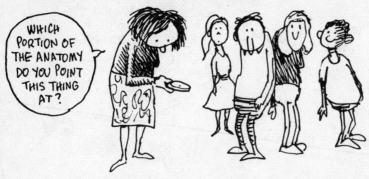

PART OF BOTH SEXES' TRADITIONAL GENDER ROLE IS TO BE ATTRACTED TO THE OTHER SEX... AND FOR MOST PEOPLE, THIS IS NO PROBLEM. THEY'RE HETEROSEXUALS, OR "STRAIGHTS"...

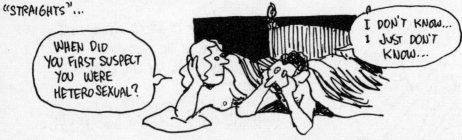

BUT EVEN STRAIGHTS MAY BE TURNED ON BY SOMEONE OF THE SAME SEX FROM TIME TO TIME. IT'S NOT UNCOMMON TO "CROSS THE LINE" JUST AS AN EXPERIMENT.

AND SOME PEOPLE "EXPERIMENT" SURPRISINGLY OFTEN WITH SAME-SEX ENCOUNTERS, WHILE RESOLUTELY THINKING OF THEMSELVES AS HETEROSEXUAL!

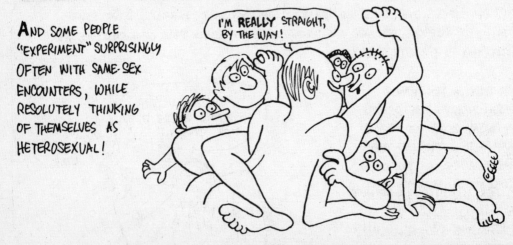

WHAT MAKES SOMEONE GAY? NOBODY KNOWS FOR SURE. MANY GAY PEOPLE REPORT THAT THEY HAVE ALWAYS "FELT GAY" AND THAT THERE WAS NO REAL CHOICE IN THE MATTER.

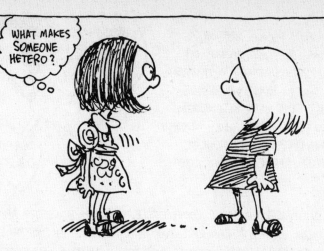

SO FAR, SCIENTIFIC RESEARCH IS INCOMPLETE BUT INTRIGUING. STUDIES OF IDENTICAL TWINS — WHO HAVE EXACTLY THE SAME GENETIC MAKEUP — SHOW THAT IF ONE TWIN IS GAY, THERE IS A 50% CHANCE THAT THE OTHER ONE IS TOO. AMONG NON-IDENTICAL TWINS OR SAME-SEX SIBLINGS, THE NUMBER IS CLOSER TO 20%. THIS STRONGLY SUGGESTS SOMETHING IN THE GENES.

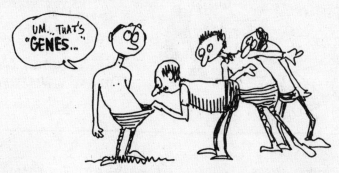

THESE RESULTS HAVE PROMPTED A SEARCH FOR "GAY GENES." RESEARCHERS HAVE FOUND A DISTINCTNE REGION ON THE X-CHROMOSOME THAT SEEMS TO BE SHARED BY GAY BROTHERS... BUT WHAT IT IS, OR WHAT IT DOES, IS ANYBODY'S GUESS AT THIS POINT. SO FAR, NOTHING HAS BEEN FOUND FOR FEMALES.

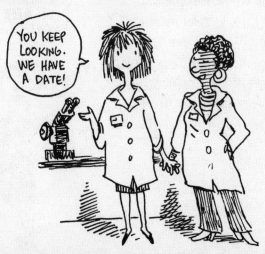

HOW MANY PEOPLE ARE GAY? THAT IS, THEY ARE MAINLY OR EXCLUSIVELY INVOLVED WITH THEIR SAME SEX? HOW CAN ANYONE KNOW? THE BEST RESEARCHERS CAN DO IS TO INTERVIEW RANDOMLY CHOSEN PEOPLE IN AN HONEST, SENSITIVE, AND CONFIDENTIAL WAY.

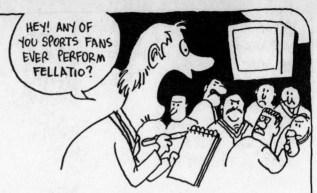

HEY! ANY OF YOU SPORTS FANS EVER PERFORM FELLATIO?

NOT MANY PEOPLE FEEL COMFORTABLE TALKING HONESTLY ABOUT THEIR SEX LIVES—ESPECIALLY WITH A STRANGER... AND THIS SUBJECT IS ONE OF THE HARDEST OF ALL... SO ANY RESEARCH RESULTS MUST BE TAKEN WITH A GRAIN OF SALT, OR MAYBE A WHOLE SALT SHAKER.

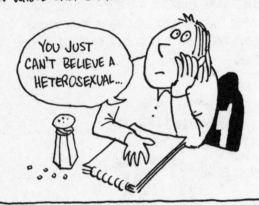

YOU JUST CAN'T BELIEVE A HETEROSEXUAL...

THE LATEST ESTIMATES ARE THAT SOMEWHERE BETWEEN 2-5% OF MEN AND AROUND 1½% OF WOMEN ARE COMPLETELY ORIENTED TOWARD HOMOSEXUALITY.

ON THE OTHER HAND, MORE WOMEN (11%) THAN MEN (7%) ARE WILLING TO ADMIT TO OCCASIONAL TWINGES OF DESIRE FOR MEMBERS OF THEIR OWN SEX — AND THAT'S ONLY THE ONES WHO ADMIT IT....

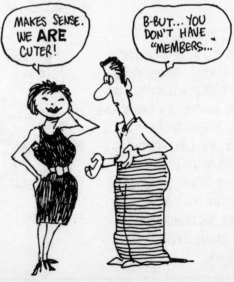

MAKES SENSE. WE **ARE** CUTER!

B-BUT... YOU DON'T HAVE "MEMBERS...

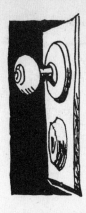

IT'S ONE THING TO ADMIT IT TO ONESELF... BUT SOMETHING ELSE TO TELL THE WORLD... SO SOME GAYS TRY TO KEEP UP HETEROSEXUAL APPEARANCES WHILE LEADING A GAY LIFE ON THE SIDE. THIS IS KNOWN AS "BEING IN THE CLOSET."

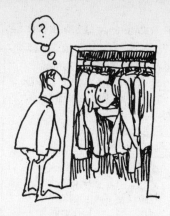

PUBLICLY ACKNOWLEDGING ONE'S HOMOSEXUALITY IS CALLED "COMING OUT."

COMING OUT TO FAMILY OFTEN CREATES A CRISIS, BUT MOST FAMILIES GRADUALLY ADJUST.

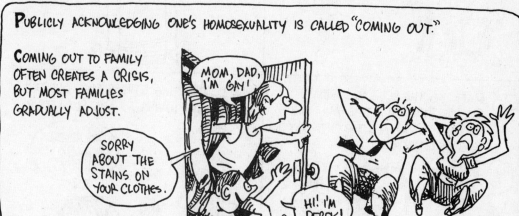

MOM, DAD, I'M GAY!

SORRY ABOUT THE STAINS ON YOUR CLOTHES.

HI! I'M DEREK!

COMING OUT TO COWORKERS AND EMPLOYERS CAN BE A BIGGER PROBLEM, ESPECIALLY FOR PEOPLE WHO WORK WITH CHILDREN, ARE IN THE MILITARY, OR HOLD POLITICAL OFFICE. SOME STAY IN THE CLOSET FOR THEIR OWN PROTECTION.

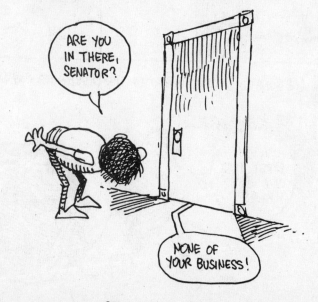

ARE YOU IN THERE, SENATOR?

NONE OF YOUR BUSINESS!

THE PROCESS OF FORMING A LESBIAN OR GAY IDENTITY HAPPENS IN STAGES.

 DISCOVERING THAT ONE'S DESIRES ARE NOT THE SAME AS MOST OTHER PEOPLE'S. THIS CAN BE CONFUSING, EVEN SCARY.

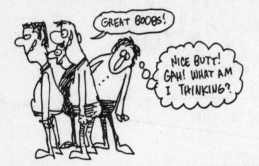

LABELING ONE'S FEELINGS AS HOMOEROTIC: THAT IS, SAME-SEX ATTRACTION AND DESIRE.

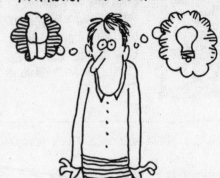

DEFINING THE SELF AS LESBIAN, GAY, OR BISEXUAL. THIS MAY NOT BE EASY, GIVEN ALL THE ANTI-GAY BIAS OUT THERE.

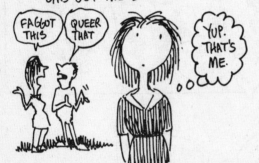

MEETING OTHERS LIKE ONESELF AND HAVING A SAME-SEX AFFAIR.

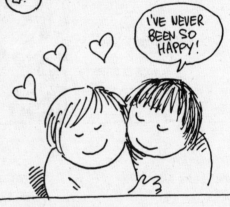

(OPTIONAL): BECOMING PART OF THE LESBIAN OR GAY SUBCULTURE.

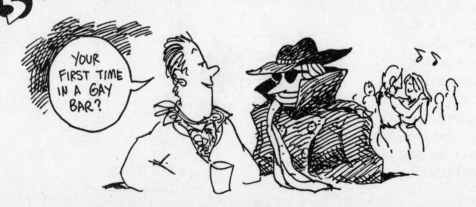

AND LET'S NOT FORGET
BISEXUALS
EITHER—PEOPLE WHO
ARE "AC-DC" OR GO
BOTH WAYS.

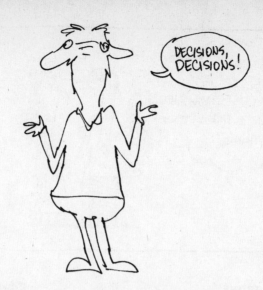

SOME BISEXUALS ARE EQUALLY ATTRACTED TO WOMEN AND MEN, WHILE OTHERS MAINLY PREFER ONE SEX OR THE OTHER. RATHER THAN SLEEPING WITH A WOMAN ONE NIGHT AND A MAN THE NEXT, ALMOST ALL BISEXUALS ARE INVOLVED IN ONE TYPE OF RELATIONSHIP FOR A PERIOD OF TIME, FOLLOWED BY THE OTHER TYPE.

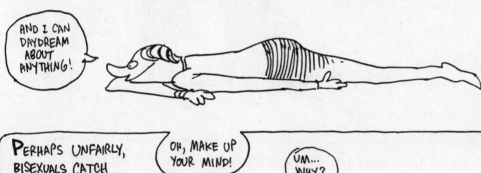

PERHAPS UNFAIRLY, BISEXUALS CATCH FLAK FROM BOTH SIDES. STRAIGHTS MAY REGARD THEM AS UNRELIABLE, WHILE GAYS MAY ACCUSE THEM OF BEING "TOURISTS" WHO WON'T COMMIT TO A GAY IDENTITY.

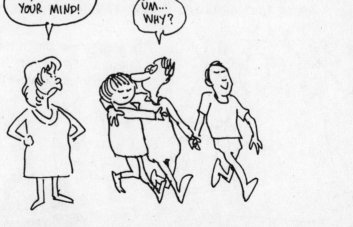

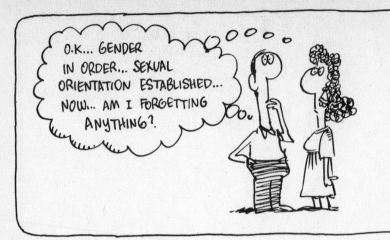

O.K.... GENDER IN ORDER... SEXUAL ORIENTATION ESTABLISHED... NOW... AM I FORGETTING ANYTHING?

For most people, the final ingredient in becoming a grown-up is finding a mate... Ms./Mr. Right... a life-partner... a soul-mate... a luv-bunny.

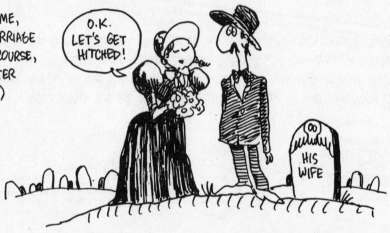

Once upon a time, this meant marriage for life. (Of course, life was shorter in those days.)

O.K. LET'S GET HITCHED!

HIS WIFE

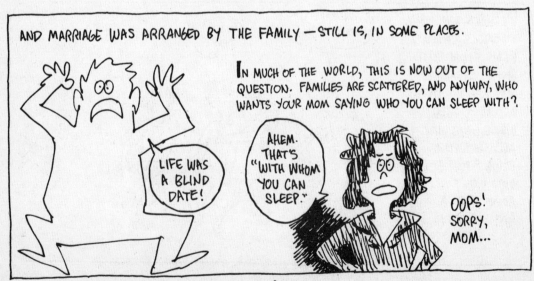

And marriage was arranged by the family — still is, in some places.

In much of the world, this is now out of the question. Families are scattered, and anyway, who wants your mom saying who you can sleep with?

LIFE WAS A BLIND DATE!

AHEM. THAT'S "WITH WHOM YOU CAN SLEEP."

OOPS! SORRY, MOM...

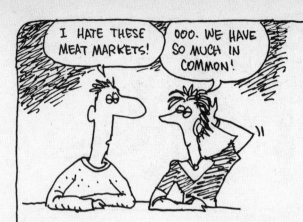

HOW DO WE MEET EACH OTHER THEN? ONE WAY IS BY CRUISING THE BARS, RESORTS, AND CLUBS CATERING TO SINGLES, WHETHER GAY OR STRAIGHT.

ANOTHER WAY WOULD BE CLASSIFIED ADS, WHERE MEN SEEK GOOD-LOOKING WOMEN AND WOMEN LOOK FOR MEN WHO ARE "SUCCESS OBJECTS." (TWO-THIRDS OF THESE ADS ARE PLACED BY MEN, BY THE WAY.)

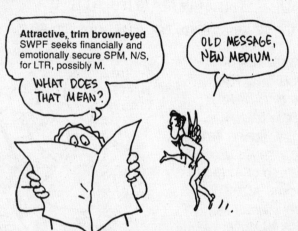

AND NOW WE HAVE ONLINE CHAT ROOMS AND COURTSHIP BY E-MAIL...

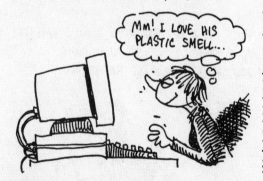

THOUGH WHEN THE CORRESPONDENTS MEET, THEY'RE OFTEN DISAPPOINTED.

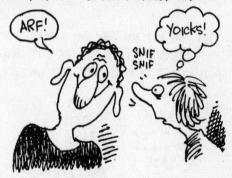

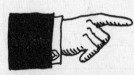

A RECENT STUDY FOUND THAT AROUND 10% OF MARRIED COUPLES AND 20% OF HETERO COUPLES "GOING TOGETHER" MET THROUGH ADS, BARS, OR ON VACATION.

THE REST, IT SEEMS, MEET IN MORE CONVENTIONAL WAYS: AT WORK AND THROUGH FRIENDS.

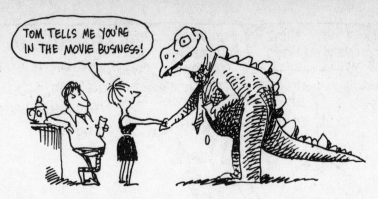

TOM TELLS ME YOU'RE IN THE MOVIE BUSINESS!

AND THEN WHAT?

ONCE THEY'VE MET, WHEN DO TWO PEOPLE JUMP INTO BED?

THE SEXES TEND TO DIFFER ON THIS POINT. WOMEN OFTEN WANT LOVE, OR AT LEAST AFFECTION, BEFORE BECOMING SEXUAL. MEN ARE MORE READY TO GO ON PHYSICAL ATTRACTION ALONE. MEN MAY VIEW SEX AS A SIMPLE PLEASURE, WHILE WOMEN TEND TO SEE IT AS A PLEASURE, BUT NOT A SIMPLE ONE (SEE CHAPTER 2)!

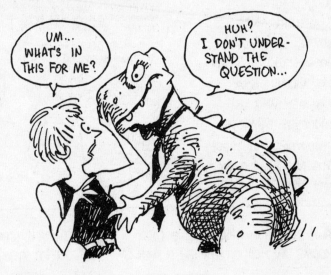

UM... WHAT'S IN THIS FOR ME?

HUH? I DON'T UNDERSTAND THE QUESTION...

THIS MAY EXPLAIN WHY GAY MEN ON AVERAGE HAVE MORE SEX PARTNERS THAN STRAIGHTS (MEN OR WOMEN). GAYS ARE NOT NECESSARILY HORNIER: IT'S JUST THAT THEIR INTENDED SEX PARTNERS ARE MALES, WHO DON'T PUT UP FEMALE RESISTANCE.

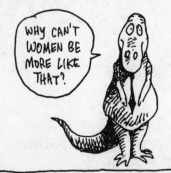

WHY CAN'T WOMEN BE MORE LIKE THAT?

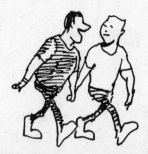

WHERE DOES OUR CULTURE STAND ON THE QUESTION OF WHEN SEX IS APPROPRIATE? THE ANSWER IS: ALL OVER THE PLACE. A SUBSTANTIAL MINORITY STILL INSIST THAT SEX IS NEVER O.K. UNLESS IT'S HETERO AND MARRIED.

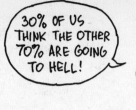
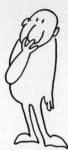

30% OF US THINK THE OTHER 70% ARE GOING TO HELL!

OTHERWISE, MOST PEOPLE WOULD PROBABLY AGREE WITH THE PROPOSITION THAT

LOVE LEGITIMIZES SEX.

THAT IS, THEY THINK SEX IS ALWAYS O.K. WITHIN A COMMITTED RELATIONSHIP, WHETHER MARRIED OR NOT. CASUAL SEX IS VIEWED AS A PROBLEM — ESPECIALLY CONSIDERING ALL THE DISEASES AND WEIRDOS OUT THERE TODAY.

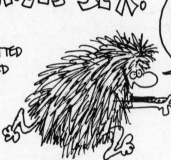

COME ON! I'VE LOVED YOU FOR THE TEN MINUTES I'VE KNOWN YOU!

YET CASUAL SEX HAPPENS... BECAUSE — LET'S FACE IT — SOMETIMES IT'S APPEALING. HERE ARE SOME

PLUSES AND MINUSES OF CASUAL SEX:

PLUSES:

* CAN BE FUN & EXCITING
* GIVES INSTANT GRATIFICATION
* PROVIDES VARIETY
* CAN BE SWEET, INTIMATE, AND MEMORABLE
* NO STRINGS

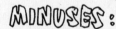

MINUSES:

* RISKY TO HEALTH AND WELL·BEING
* CAN GROW BORING AND POINTLESS
* CAN BECOME COMPULSIVE & NO FUN
* CAN INTERFERE WITH THE CAPACITY TO FORM LASTING RELATIONSHIPS
* CAN BREAK UP A PRIMARY RELATIONSHIP
* CAN BE SOCIALLY STIGMATIZING (ESPECIALLY FOR WOMEN)
* PARTNER'S NAME MAY BE FORGOTTEN AT CRITICAL MOMENT.

To MOST OF US, THE CONS WIN: SURVEYS SHOW THAT MOST PEOPLE BELIEVE THE BEST SEXUAL EXPERIENCES HAPPEN IN MEANINGFUL RELATIONSHIPS.

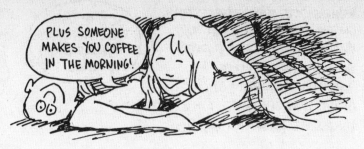

AND BY THE WAY, GAY MEN AND WOMEN ARE JUST AS INTERESTED AS THEIR STRAIGHT COUNTERPARTS IN RELATIONSHIPS BASED ON LOVE AND AFFECTION. IN FACT, ENTERING A LOVING RELATIONSHIP WITH A MEMBER OF THE SAME SEX IS AN IMPORTANT STEP IN ESTABLISHING A LESBIAN OR GAY IDENTITY.

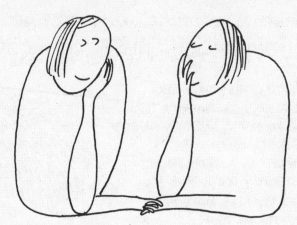

So WHILE WE'RE AT IT, LET'S LIST SOME

PROS AND CONS OF COMMITTED SEX

PROS:

* SAFER
* SIMPLIFIES NEGOTIATION
* CAN BUILD PHYSICAL FULFILLMENT, AS PARTNERS LEARN EACH OTHERS' PREFERENCES
* CAN BUILD LONG-TERM EMOTIONAL FULFILLMENT
* CAN PROVIDE A SETTING FOR SEXUAL EXPLORATION
* CAN MAKE BABIES, IF WANTED
* SOCIALLY ACCEPTABLE

CONS:

* SAME OLD, SAME OLD
* INTENSITY AND FREQUENCY LIKELY TO FADE
* MAY OVERSIMPLIFY NEGOTIATION

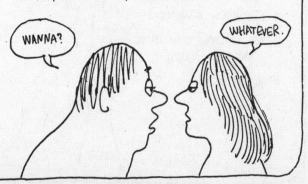

So we enter relationships. We "go together," seeing each other more or less exclusively while living apart.

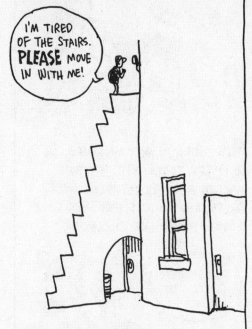

I'm tired of the stairs. **PLEASE** move in with me!

Or we **COHABIT**, living together without getting married. Cohabitation has risen by 500% since 1970 in the U.S.A. About half of all young Americans will have cohabited with someone by age 30.

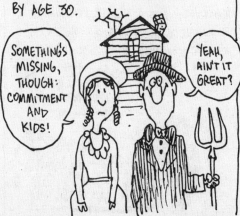

Something's missing, though: commitment and kids!

Yeah, ain't it great?

Cohabitation is so common now that some cities and companies now recognize **DOMESTIC PARTNERSHIP** as a quasi-legal union. Domestic partners may register and receive the same insurance benefits or pension coverage as spouses.

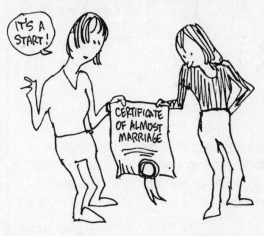

It's a start!

CERTIFICATE OF ALMOST MARRIAGE

Among heterosexuals, cohabitation rarely lasts longer than two years. The couple either breaks up or gets married.

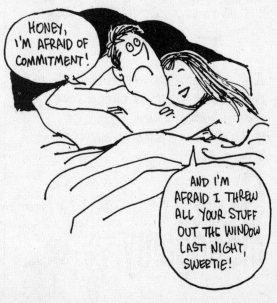

Honey, I'm afraid of commitment!

And I'm afraid I threw all your stuff out the window last night, sweetie!

95

AND THEN THERE'S GOOD OLD MARRIAGE, THE LONG-TERM-COMMITMENT-IN-PUBLIC THING. FOR GAYS, THIS IS STILL NOT A LEGAL OPTION, OWING TO OPPOSITION FROM THE UPHOLDERS OF TRADITIONAL VALUES.

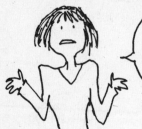

WHEN WE TRY TO FORM FAMILIES, THEY CALL US ANTI-FAMILY!

FOR HETEROS, MARRIAGE IS CHANGING. TO BEGIN WITH, IT'S STARTING LATER: AT AGE 24½ FOR WOMEN AND 26½ FOR MEN, ON AVERAGE.

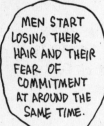

MEN START LOSING THEIR HAIR AND THEIR FEAR OF COMMITMENT AT AROUND THE SAME TIME.

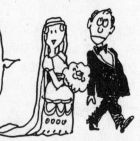

AND IT ENDS SOONER: ABOUT 50-60% OF NEW MARRIAGES END IN DIVORCE, AND THE AVERAGE MARRIAGE NOW LASTS JUST 7 YEARS. THIS SYSTEM OF MARRYING ONE AFTER ANOTHER IS CALLED

Serial monogamy.

WHAT DO YOU CALL IT WHEN YOU ONLY EAT CORNFLAKES?

CEREAL MONOTONY?

WHAT ABOUT SEX IN MARRIAGE?

SEX IN MARRIAGE... WHAT'S THAT?

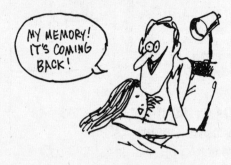

IT'S TRUE... IN MOST MARRIAGES, WE DO IT LESS OFTEN AS TIME PASSES. MARRIED MEN'S TESTOSTERONE LEVEL DROOPS, AND SO DOES THEIR SEX DRIVE — THOUGH NOT TO ZERO!

MY MEMORY! IT'S COMING BACK!

BUT BEFORE YOU START TO CRY, CONSIDER THIS: LESS-FREQUENT SEX IS NOT NECESSARILY EXPERIENCED NEGATIVELY, AND A HIGHER PERCENTAGE OF MARRIEDS THAN SINGLES REPORT SATISFACTION WITH THEIR SEX LIVES.

THESE POLLSTERS ARE EVERYWHERE!

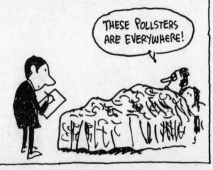

How faithful are we to our spouses? It seems to be true that cheating is more common in bad marriages. One biological factor is that arguing drives up testosterone levels!

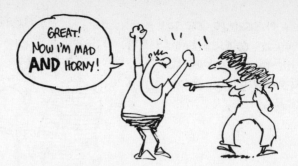

GREAT! NOW I'M MAD **AND** HORNY!

Some statistics: Recent surveys have found that 21-25% of men and 11-15% of women have cheated. Among younger couples, age 22 to 33, 7% of men and **12%** of women admit to being unfaithful.

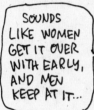

SOUNDS LIKE WOMEN GET IT OVER WITH EARLY, AND MEN KEEP AT IT...

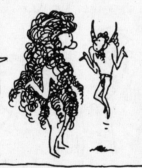

Discovering a mate's infidelity usually creates a crisis in the relationship!

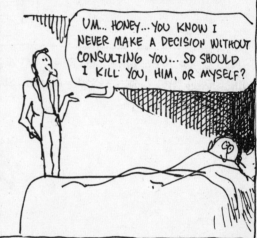

UM... HONEY... YOU KNOW I NEVER MAKE A DECISION WITHOUT CONSULTING YOU... SO SHOULD I KILL YOU, HIM, OR MYSELF?

Some couples can tolerate an "open marriage" with some amount of outside sex. Gay men seem to tolerate this better than heterosexuals.

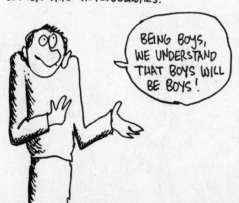

BEING BOYS, WE UNDERSTAND THAT BOYS WILL BE BOYS!

And around 2% of Americans have some experience with "swinging" or mate-swapping. Contrary to popular opinion, swingers tend to be politically conservative, white, and middle-class.

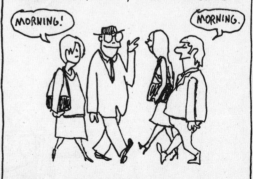

MORNING!

MORNING.

IF A CRISIS DOES LEAD TO
DIVORCE, COUPLES USUALLY
FIND NEW PARTNERS AND
REMARRY WITHIN FOUR
YEARS.

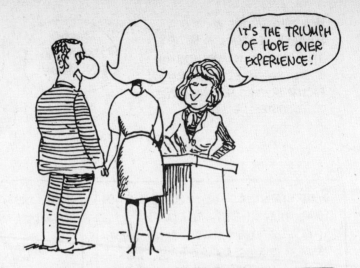

IT'S THE TRIUMPH
OF HOPE OVER
EXPERIENCE!

AND SO WE AGE... HAVE CHILDREN... WATCH THEM GROW... AND WE SUFFER LOSS —
INCLUDING THE LOSS OF SOME OF OUR SEXUAL RESPONSE...BUT MOST PEOPLE NEVER
LOSE INTEREST IN SEX!

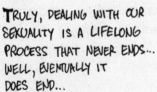

UNFORTUNATELY!

TRULY, DEALING WITH OUR
SEXUALITY IS A LIFELONG
PROCESS THAT NEVER ENDS...
WELL, EVENTUALLY IT
DOES END...

GRANDMA, CAN
NECROPHILIA
EVER HAPPEN BY
MUTUAL CONSENT?

READ MY
WILL!

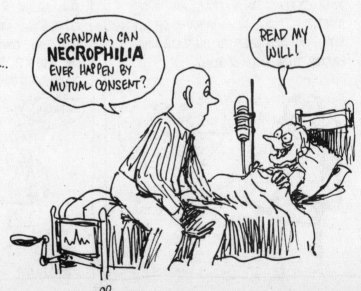

·CHAPTER 6·
COMMUNICATION

COMMUNICATION IS AN ESSENTIAL PART OF SEXUALITY. ANIMALS SIGNAL THEIR INTEREST IN SEX WITH AN ASSORTMENT OF SMELLS, SONGS, AND VISUAL CUES. PEOPLE ARE MORE SUBTLE. WE WEAR COLOGNE OR PERFUME, PUT ON CERTAIN CLOTHES AND MAKE-UP, USE OUR EYES, SMILES, POSTURE, AND HAIR — AND DON'T FORGET OUR WORDS!

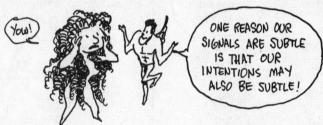

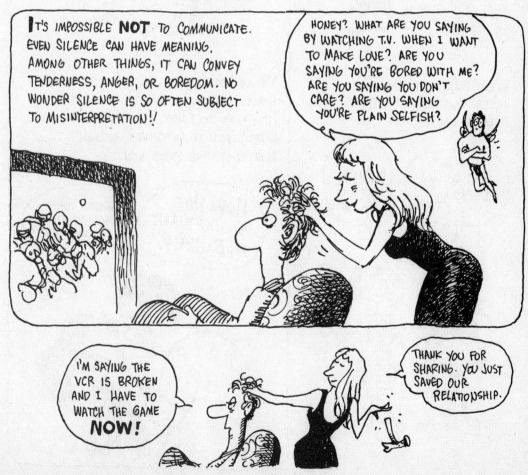

When we meet a potential partner, we send out **FLIRTING** signals: eye contact, smiles, teasing, light touching, etc...

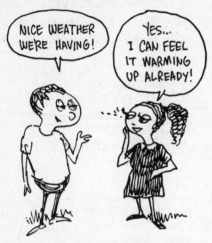

With flirtation, what we say matters less than how we say it.

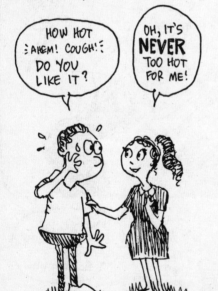

Unfortunately, a certain amount of misunderstanding results from the fact that women and men have somewhat different flirting styles.

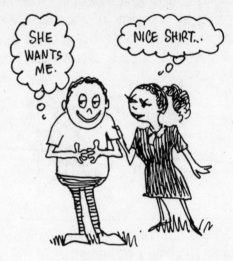

Women may flirt just for fun, without really intending to go any farther... Men tend to flirt with overt sexual intent and to interpret women's flirtation the same way.

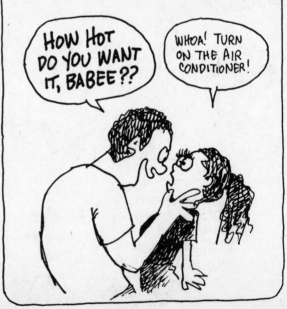

100

WOMEN ALSO TEND TO BE MORE INDIRECT THAN MEN. WHEN A WOMAN FLIRTS, SHE MAY SHOW INTEREST BY THE MOST SUBTLE SIGNS: MAKING MOMENTARY EYE CONTACT, MOVING SLIGHTLY CLOSER, OR JUST FLIPPING HER HAIR. MEN MAY MISS THESE SIGNALS COMPLETELY.

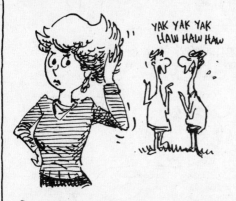

YAK YAK YAK HAW HAW HAW

A MAN IS MORE LIKELY TO MOVE IN CLOSE AND DELIVER AN "OPENING LINE."

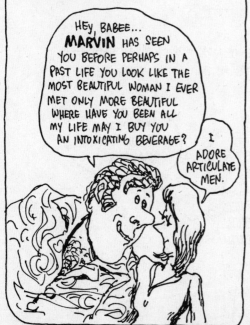

HEY, BABEE... MARVIN HAS SEEN YOU BEFORE PERHAPS IN A PAST LIFE YOU LOOK LIKE THE MOST BEAUTIFUL WOMAN I EVER MET ONLY MORE BEAUTIFUL WHERE HAVE YOU BEEN ALL MY LIFE MAY I BUY YOU AN INTOXICATING BEVERAGE?

I ADORE ARTICULATE MEN.

GUYS, TAKE NOTE! PLEASE!! WOMEN PREFER AN INNOCUOUS OPENER TO A BLUNT ONE.

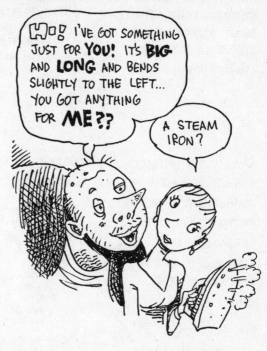

HO! I'VE GOT SOMETHING JUST FOR YOU! IT'S BIG AND LONG AND BENDS SLIGHTLY TO THE LEFT... YOU GOT ANYTHING FOR ME??

A STEAM IRON?

BY THE WAY, IF A WOMAN OPENS THE CONVERSATION, MEN TEND TO BE THRILLED, NO MATTER WHAT SHE SAYS!

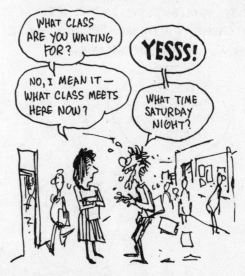

WHAT CLASS ARE YOU WAITING FOR?

NO, I MEAN IT — WHAT CLASS MEETS HERE NOW?

YESSS!

WHAT TIME SATURDAY NIGHT?

When lesbians and gay men meet someone of interest, they face a problem most straights don't even think about: whether the person shares their sexual orientation.

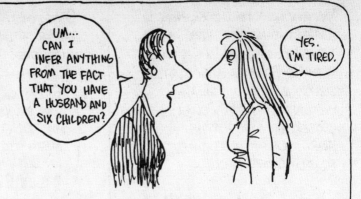

Unless the introduction is through friends or happens at a gay gathering place, they may have to rely on "GAY-DAR." Mannerisms, speech patterns, cultural references, and lingering glances are some of the clues.

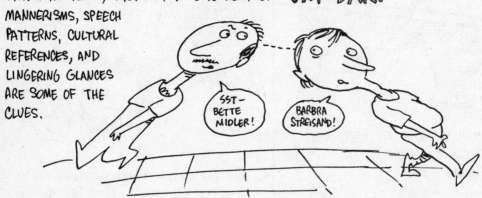

Note: Prolonged eye contact between straight men — or chimpanzees! — is perceived as a threat. Between gay men, it's an invitation. Talk about grounds for misunderstanding!!!

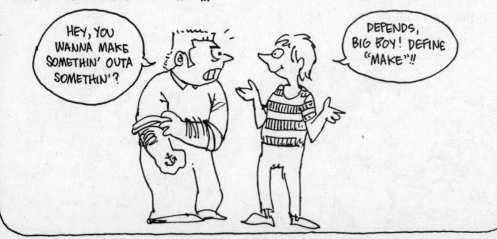

LIKE HETERO MALES, A GAY MALE IS MORE LIKELY THAN A FEMALE TO INITIATE SEXUAL ACTIVITY EARLY IN A RELATIONSHIP — AND MORE LIKELY THAN A HETERO MALE TO HAVE HIS INTEREST PROMPTLY REQUITED.

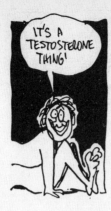

ON THE OTHER HAND, THE EXPECTATION THAT GUYS ARE ALWAYS READY TO GO CAN MAKE IT HARDER FOR A GAY MALE TO SAY NO.

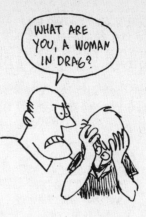

SOME LESBIANS MAY FIND IT HARD TO MEET OTHERS AND START A RELATIONSHIP, BECAUSE AS WOMEN THEY ARE LESS COMFORTABLE MAKING THE FIRST MOVE.

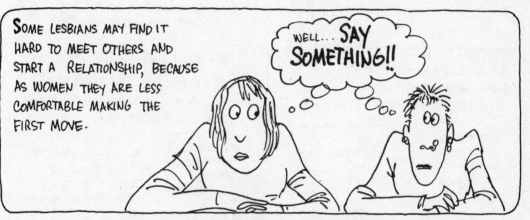

LESBIANS TEND TO RELY MORE ON FRIENDS FOR INTRODUCTIONS.

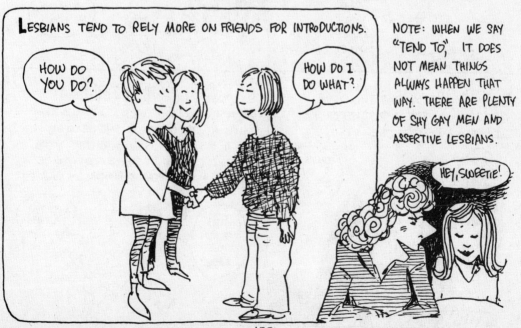

NOTE: WHEN WE SAY "TEND TO", IT DOES NOT MEAN THINGS ALWAYS HAPPEN THAT WAY. THERE ARE PLENTY OF SHY GAY MEN AND ASSERTIVE LESBIANS.

BEFORE EMBARKING ON A SEXUAL VOYAGE, WE OWE IT TO OUR POTENTIAL PARTNER (AND OURSELVES!) TO HAVE

THE CONVERSATION.

IT'S NOT AN EASY CONVERSATION, BUT IT IS IMPORTANT, AND IT'S GUARANTEED TO INCREASE THE LEVEL OF INTIMACY IN YOUR RELATIONSHIP.

UM... WE HAVE TO TALK... AND TALK... AND TALK...

:GROAN: I KNOW IT!

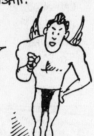

OR END IT ON THE SPOT, IN WHICH CASE YOU'RE BETTER OFF WITHOUT THE TURKEY, BELIEVE ME!

HERE ARE THE TOPICS THAT NEED DISCUSSING: ↓

INTENTION: WHAT DOES SEXUAL INVOLVEMENT MEAN TO YOU? LOVE? COMMITMENT? EXERCISE?

WHAT IF I SAID I WON'T KNOW UNTIL IT'S OVER?

I'D SAY YOU WERE MORE HONEST THAN MANY!

CONTRACEPTION & CONDOMS: THERE HAS TO BE MUTUAL AGREEMENT ON THESE EARLY ENOUGH TO ALLOW FOR PREPARATION.

SEE CHAPTER 9 FOR DETAILS!

AT THE VERY LEAST, BRING A CONDOM AND BE PREPARED TO BACK UP YOUR CONVICTIONS WITH ACTION!

NO GLOVE, NO LOVE!

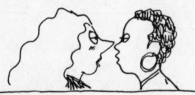

STDs: YOU MUST TELL YOUR PARTNER IF YOU HAVE A DISEASE OR HAVE EVER BEEN EXPOSED TO ONE.

UM... UM... UM... I HAD MEASLES WHEN I WAS 7...

THAT'S A "D," BUT IT'S NOT "S.T."!

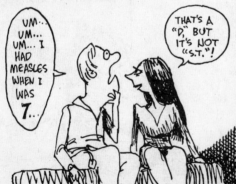

SEXUAL ACTIVITIES: OBVIOUSLY, YOU CAN'T COVER ABSOLUTELY EVERYTHING AT THE OUTSET OF A RELATIONSHIP... BUT IF ONE PERSON IS UNCOMFORTABLE DOING SOMETHING, SHE OR HE SHOULD FEEL FREE TO SPEAK UP WITHOUT FEAR OF RIDICULE OR COERCION.

CHAINS, BUT NO WHIPS, PLEASE!

NOW YOU TELL ME!

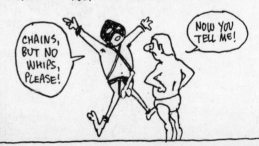

IF YOU ARE INITIATING SEXUAL ACTIVITY, YOU SHOULD BE SURE THAT THE OTHER PERSON WANTS IT... BUT DON'T WORRY! ASKING PERMISSION CAN BE VERY SEXY...

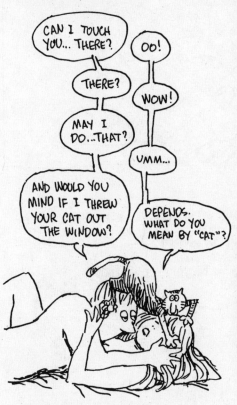

CAN I TOUCH YOU... THERE?

THERE?

MAY I DO...THAT?

AND WOULD YOU MIND IF I THREW YOUR CAT OUT THE WINDOW?

OO!

WOW!

UMM...

DEPENDS. WHAT DO YOU MEAN BY "CAT"?

BUT SOMETIMES, ALL IS NOT AGREEABLE... WHICH BRINGS UP A BIG, IMPORTANT, HEADLINE-TYPE TOPIC...

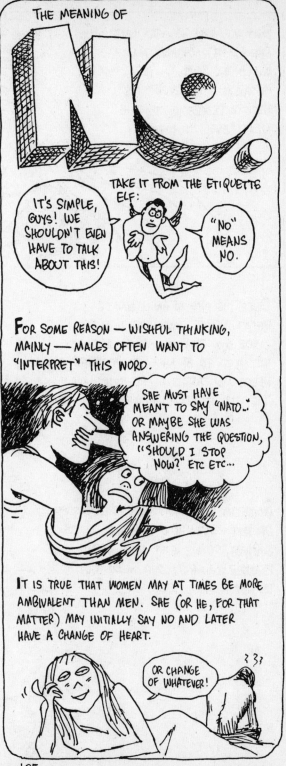

THE MEANING OF

NO.

TAKE IT FROM THE ETIQUETTE ELF:

IT'S SIMPLE, GUYS! WE SHOULDN'T EVEN HAVE TO TALK ABOUT THIS!

"NO" MEANS NO.

FOR SOME REASON — WISHFUL THINKING, MAINLY — MALES OFTEN WANT TO "INTERPRET" THIS WORD.

SHE MUST HAVE MEANT TO SAY "NATO"... OR MAYBE SHE WAS ANSWERING THE QUESTION, "SHOULD I STOP NOW?" ETC ETC...

IT IS TRUE THAT WOMEN MAY AT TIMES BE MORE AMBIVALENT THAN MEN. SHE (OR HE, FOR THAT MATTER) MAY INITIALLY SAY NO AND LATER HAVE A CHANGE OF HEART.

OR CHANGE OF WHATEVER!

BUT YOU WILL HAVE TO WAIT UNTIL SHE (OR HE) ACTUALLY AND WILLINGLY SAYS "MAYBE," "SOON," "COAX ME," OR EVEN "YES" BEFORE PROCEEDING TO THE NEXT LEVEL OF INTIMACY.

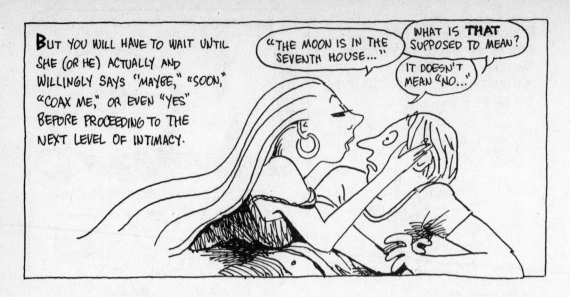

ONCE WE ARE IN AN INTIMATE RELATIONSHIP, COMMUNICATION CAN HELP GUIDE OUR ONGOING SEXUAL ACTIVITY. WE NEED TO BE ABLE TO DESCRIBE OUR NEEDS AND TASTES IN ORDER TO HAVE THE KIND OF SEX LIFE WE WANT.

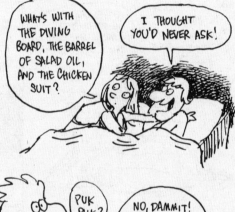

SOMETIMES WE MAY FEEL EMBARRASSED, OR NOT KNOW HOW TO BRING UP THE SUBJECT, SO WE JUST HOPE OUR PARTNER CAN READ OUR MIND. THIS IS NOT A GOOD IDEA.

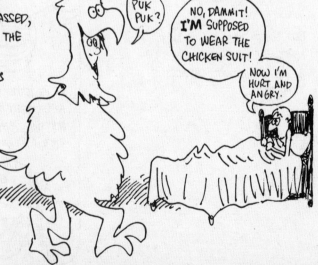

ONE THING THAT HELPS IN TALKING ABOUT SEX IS TO USE THE RIGHT VOCABULARY. THIS CAN BE AWKWARD AT FIRST. SOME WORDS SOUND CLINICAL AND COLD, WHILE OTHERS ARE NOT SPOKEN IN POLITE COMPANY, OR AREN'T SUPPOSED TO BE...

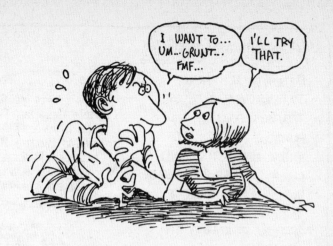

IT HELPS TO LEARN WHAT EVERYTHING IS ACTUALLY CALLED (FOR EXAMPLE, THE VAGINA IS THE INSIDE PART; THE VULVA IS THE OUTSIDE PART), SO AT LEAST WE CAN MAKE OURSELVES UNDERSTOOD! IN TIME, WE FIND OUT WHAT TERMS OUR PARTNER PREFERS.

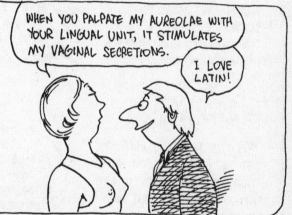

ONCE A LEVEL OF TRUST IS ESTABLISHED, PARTNERS MAY FEEL COMFORTABLE — MORE THAN COMFORTABLE, **AROUSED** — SPOUTING ALL KINDS OF EROTIC TALK. WHO KNOWS, THEY MAY INVENT SOME OF THEIR OWN!

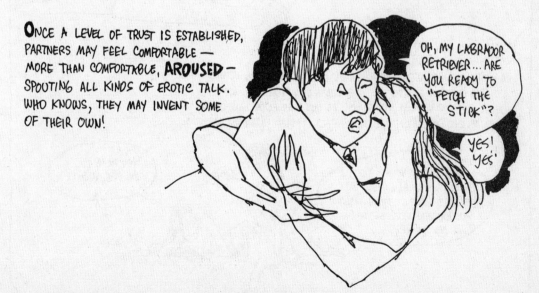

SELF-DISCLOSURE:

OFTEN, WE ARE AFRAID TO REVEAL OUR INNERMOST THOUGHTS, FEELINGS, AND FANTASIES... MAYBE, WE THINK, OUR PARTNER WILL LAUGH... CRY... BE REPELLED OR HURT. IN FACT, MOST OF THE TIME, A PARTNER IS GRATEFUL AT HEARING THE DEEP STUFF, AND THIS ACCEPTANCE DRAWS PEOPLE CLOSER. BESIDES, SHARING OUR THOUGHTS ENCOURAGES A PARTNER TO DO THE SAME!

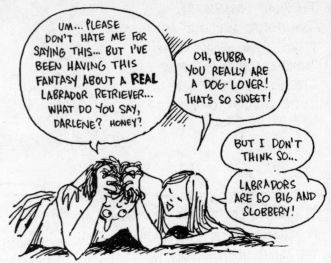

FEEDBACK:

WHEN WE LISTEN, IT HELPS TO LET THE OTHER PERSON KNOW THAT WE UNDERSTAND (OR ARE TRYING TO UNDERSTAND) WHAT HE OR SHE IS SAYING.

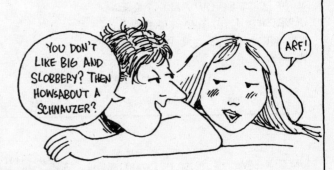

CONGRUENCE: THIS MEANS

AGREEMENT BETWEEN THE MESSAGE AND THE MEANING BEHIND IT. THE ACTUAL WORDS WE USE SHOULD MATCH OUR TONE OF VOICE, OUR VOLUME AND PITCH, AS WELL AS BODY LANGUAGE SUCH AS EYE CONTACT, PHYSICAL CONTACT, FACIAL EXPRESSIONS, ETC.

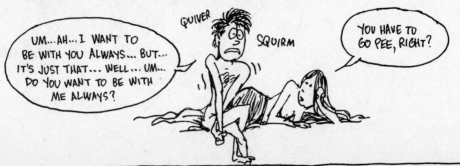

108

No matter how much we love and desire each other, eventually we are bound to run into some kind of problem or conflict in our sex lives. One wants sex and the other doesn't... one wants a particular act, the other doesn't... one can't get it up, the other can't keep it down...

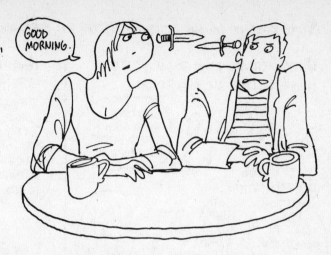

When our sex lives get difficult, the first thing we need to figure out is what the problem really is. Is it a question of actual desire or sexual function? Or an "unrelated" problem elsewhere in the relationship, like money, attention, housework, or jealousy?

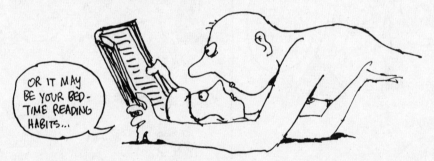

Or it could even be a problem outside the relationship, like politics or problems at work.

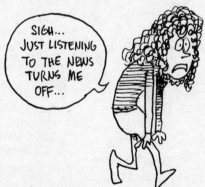

SOME KINDS OF COMMUNICATION ARE BETTER FOR RESOLVING CONFLICTS THAN OTHERS.

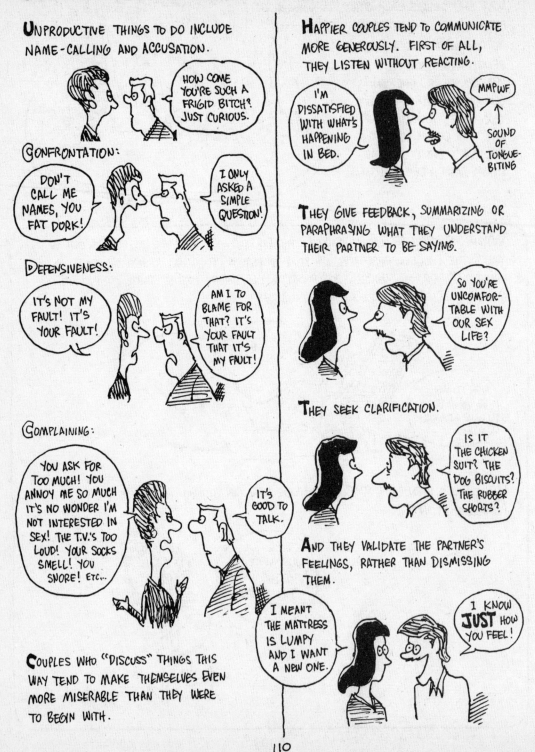

UNPRODUCTIVE THINGS TO DO INCLUDE NAME-CALLING AND ACCUSATION.

CONFRONTATION:

DEFENSIVENESS:

COMPLAINING:

COUPLES WHO "DISCUSS" THINGS THIS WAY TEND TO MAKE THEMSELVES EVEN MORE MISERABLE THAN THEY WERE TO BEGIN WITH.

HAPPIER COUPLES TEND TO COMMUNICATE MORE GENEROUSLY. FIRST OF ALL, THEY LISTEN WITHOUT REACTING.

THEY GIVE FEEDBACK, SUMMARIZING OR PARAPHRASING WHAT THEY UNDERSTAND THEIR PARTNER TO BE SAYING.

THEY SEEK CLARIFICATION.

AND THEY VALIDATE THE PARTNER'S FEELINGS, RATHER THAN DISMISSING THEM.

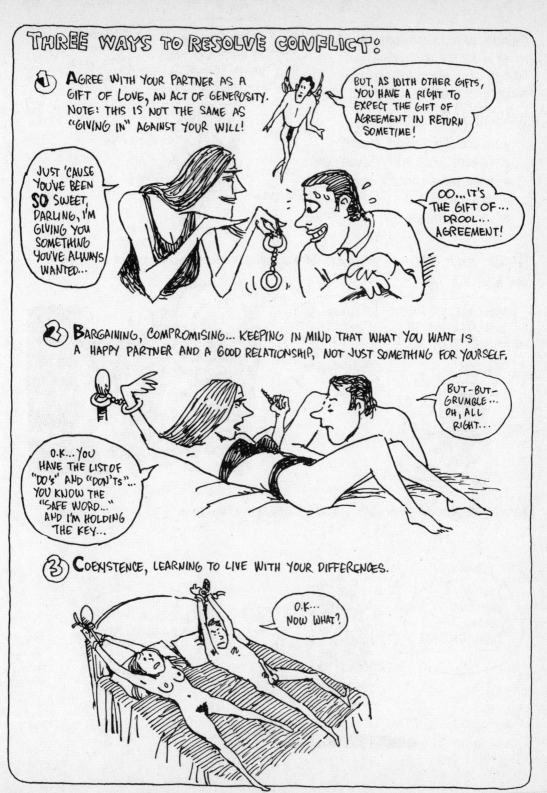

FINALLY, IN SUCCESSFUL COMMUNICATION AS IN SO MUCH ELSE, TIMING IS EVERYTHING. GOOD TIMES TO TALK ABOUT HIGHLY CHARGED SEXUAL ISSUES **DO NOT** INCLUDE:

* IN BED AFTER YOU'VE STARTED
* IN BED, JUST AFTER YOU'VE FINISHED
* WHEN YOU'RE LATE FOR SOMETHING
* JUST BEFORE A JOB INTERVIEW OR FINAL EXAM
* ON VALENTINE'S DAY

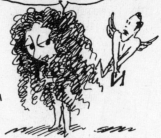

TALKING ABOUT SEX CAN BE DIFFICULT. IT REQUIRES PATIENCE, TENDERNESS, TOTAL ATTENTION, AND ADEQUATE TIME.

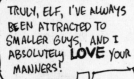

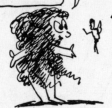

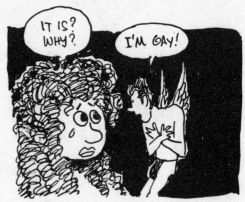

IN THE END, EVEN IF IT DOESN'T WORK — WASN'T IT WORTH A TRY?

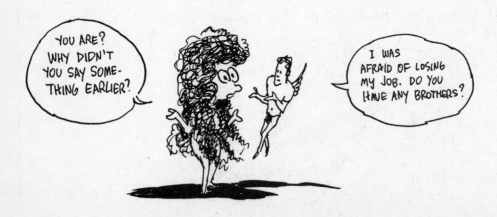

CHAPTER 7
♡ ♡ ♡ LOVE ♡ ♡ ♡

AN EMOTION OF THE HEART AND OTHER PORTIONS OF THE ANATOMY

> JUST FOR ONCE, CAN'T THERE BE A SEX BOOK WITHOUT A CHAPTER ON LOVE?

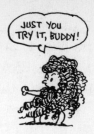

> JUST YOU TRY IT, BUDDY!

I'T'S A STRANGE FACT THAT WHEN WE WISH TO SPEAK ABOUT SEXUAL ACTS, OUR CHOICES ARE LIMITED. WE CAN EITHER USE WORDS THAT ARE BLUNT AND UGLY ("BOINK, HUMP, SCREW"), LATINATE MEDICAL TERMINOLOGY ("COITUS, FELLATIO"), OR CREATIVE EUPHEMISMS.

> LET'S "LET THE CHICKEN OUT OF THE COOP."

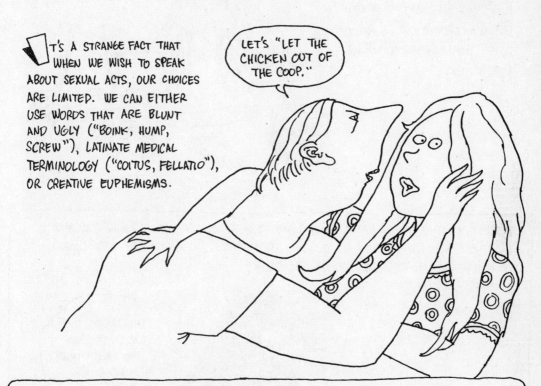

THERE IS ONLY ONE SYNONYM FOR SEX THAT REALLY SOUNDS SWEET, AND THAT'S "MAKING LOVE."

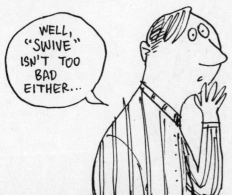

> WELL, "SWIVE" ISN'T TOO BAD EITHER...

WHAT IS THIS THING CALLED LOVE, ANYWAY?

Can animals love each other? It's hard to say. When mating is a brief encounter, they probably do not feel love, at least not for long. The female praying mantis, for example, which bites off her mate's head during copulation, surely loves him longer than he loves her...

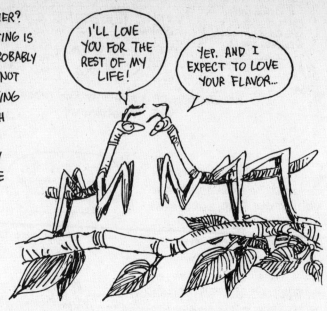

People, on the other hand, form long-term pairs. We need powerful and lasting emotions to cement our relationships. You might say that love is nature's glue for holding us together.

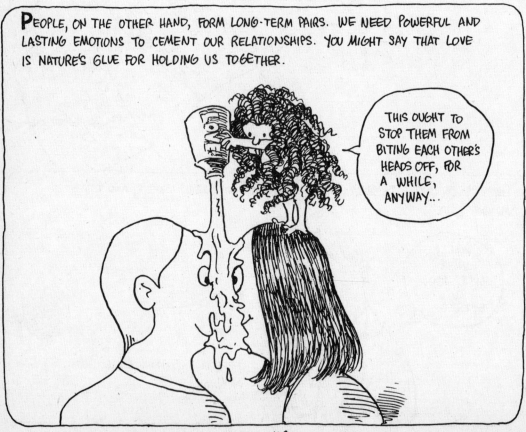

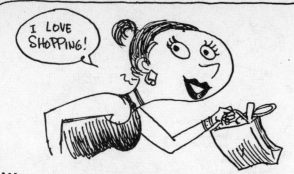

But wait, you say, if love is about merging genes, then what about the other kinds of love we hear about: brotherly love, love of God, love of country, etc.?

Well... there is a connection. All love is an emotional attachment to someone or something else. Religious ecstasy is famous for its erotic component, especially when the devotees remain celibate, like catholic nuns, who are sometimes called the "brides of christ."

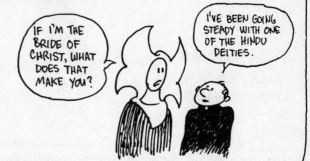

In fact, some would argue that the flame of love burns hottest when physical union with the beloved is impossible. Maybe, in an era of easy sex, erotic feeling isn't as intense as it used to be.

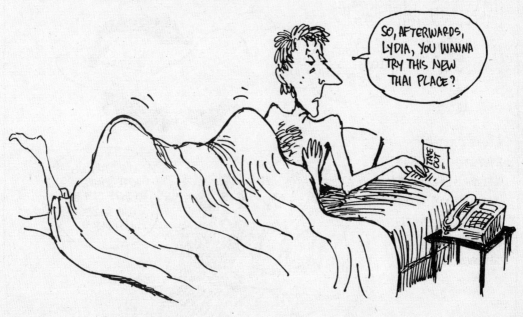

How do we fall in love? No matter how we first make contact with someone, we seem to need face-to-face contact to be sure there is physical attraction. For most of us,

LUST

is a key component of love, especially at the beginning.

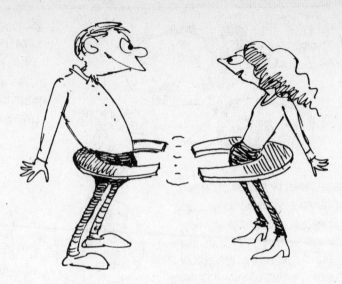

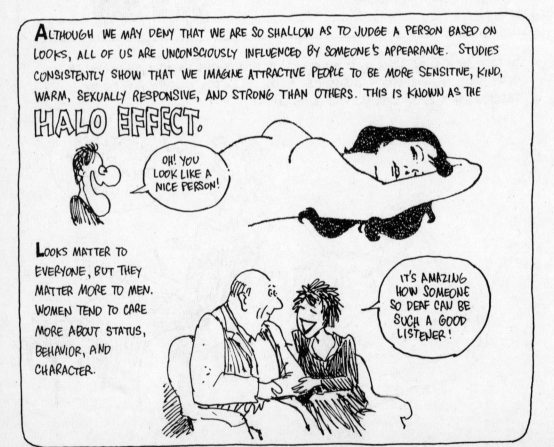

Although we may deny that we are so shallow as to judge a person based on looks, all of us are unconsciously influenced by someone's appearance. Studies consistently show that we imagine attractive people to be more sensitive, kind, warm, sexually responsive, and strong than others. This is known as the

HALO EFFECT.

Oh! You look like a nice person!

Looks matter to everyone, but they matter more to men. Women tend to care more about status, behavior, and character.

It's amazing how someone so deaf can be such a good listener!

WHAT ABOUT LOVE AT FIRST SIGHT? OF COURSE, IT CAN'T REALLY BE LOVE, IF WE DON'T KNOW THE OTHER PERSON, BUT WE CAN STILL BECOME AROUSED, INFATUATED, OR OBSESSED AFTER A BRIEF ENCOUNTER. THIS FEELING, ASIDE FROM BEING ALL-CONSUMING, IS ALSO USUALLY UNREQUITED.

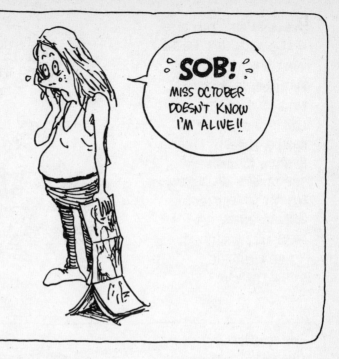

WE MIGHT ALSO MENTION LOVE AT FIRST SMELL. SOME SCIENTISTS SUSPECT THAT PEOPLE, LIKE MOTHS, MAY EXUDE SUBTLY SCENTED CHEMICALS, OR PHEROMONES, THAT TRIGGER SEXUAL DESIRE. WE ARE SUPPOSEDLY UNAWARE OF THESE AROMAS, DESPITE THEIR POWERFUL EFFECT.

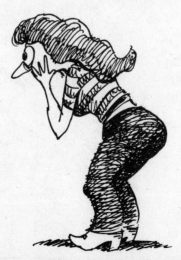

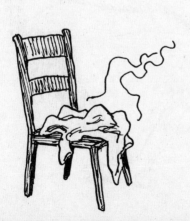

BESIDES LUST, WHAT ELSE IS LOVE MADE OF? WE CAN NAME SOME OF THE FEELINGS WE ASSOCIATE WITH LOVE AND THE LOVED ONE: TRUST, CARING, HONESTY, LIKING, RESPECT, CONCERN FOR THE OTHER'S WELL-BEING, LOYALTY, ACCEPTANCE, SUPPORTIVENESS, AND ABOVE ALL, WANTING TO BE WITH THE OTHER PERSON...

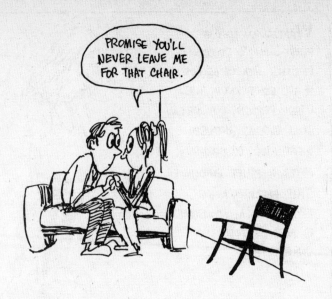

AND BEHAVIORS LIKE VERBAL EXPRESSIONS OF LOVE, SELF-DISCLOSURE, GIVING PRESENTS, DOING FAVORS, HUGS, KISSES, FOOT MASSAGES — AND NOT LEAST, PUTTING UP WITH THE OTHER PERSON'S PECULIARITIES.

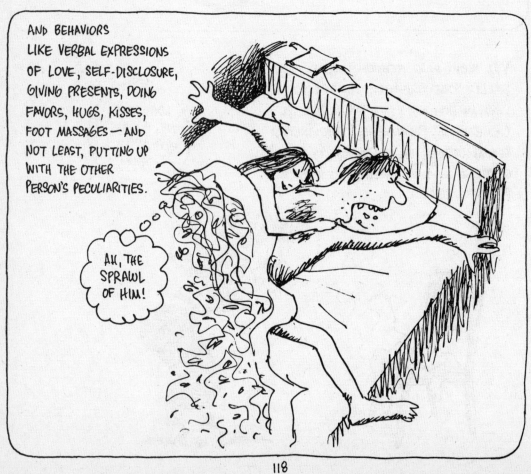

ASIDE FROM THE LUST, LOVE SOUNDS A LOT LIKE FRIENDSHIP. IN FACT, FRIENDSHIP AND LOVE SHARE MANY QUALITIES: COMPANIONSHIP, ACCEPTANCE, FORGIVENESS, RESPECT, LOYALTY, TRUST, ETC... DOES LOVE HAVE ANY OTHER INGREDIENTS BESIDES FRIENDSHIP AND LUST??

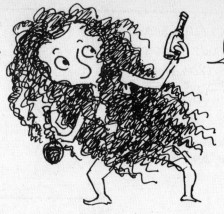

HM... BETRAYAL? NO... DECEPTION? NO...

FOR A RELATIONSHIP TO ENDURE, IT NEEDS THE C-WORD: **COMMITMENT.** THE PLEDGE TO STICK WITH IT THROUGH GOOD TIMES AND BAD IS ESSENTIAL TO FAMILY STABILITY.

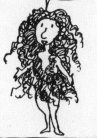

ISN'T THIS WHAT MARRIAGE IS ABOUT?

ANOTHER INGREDIENT WOULD BE **EXCLUSIVITY.** WE EXPECT OUR LOVER TO BE FAITHFUL.

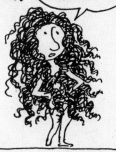

YOUR FRIEND CAN HAVE OTHER FRIENDS, BUT YOUR LOVER — ?

SO MAYBE THAT'S OUR FORMULA:

LUST + FRIENDSHIP + COMMITMENT + EXCLUSIVITY = LOVE.

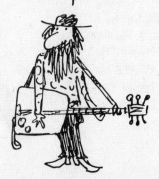

WELL, THAT'S SOLVED. NOW WE CAN STOP WRITING SONGS ABOUT IT!

OF COURSE, YOU CAN'T REALLY REDUCE LOVE TO A FORMULA, BUT THAT HASN'T STOPPED SOME PSYCHOLOGISTS FROM TRYING! **ROBERT STERNBERG,** FOR EXAMPLE, SEES LOVE AS A TRIANGLE WITH THREE COMPONENTS: INTIMACY, PASSION, AND COMMITMENT.

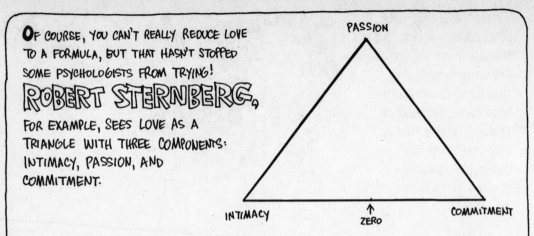

THE IDEAL, WHICH STERNBERG CALLS CONSUMMATE LOVE, IS HIGH IN ALL THREE COMPONENTS AND LOOKS LIKE THE FIRST TRIANGLE ON THE PAGE. OTHER TRIANGLES ARE ALSO POSSIBLE.

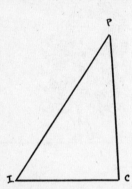

ROMANTIC LOVE: HIGH PASSION, HIGH INTIMACY, LOW COMMITMENT

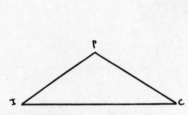

COMPANIONATE LOVE: HIGH INTIMACY AND COMMITMENT, LOW PASSION

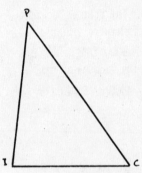

FATUOUS OR DECEPTIVE LOVE: HIGH PASSION AND COMMITMENT, LOW INTIMACY

EACH PERSON BRINGS A TRIANGLE TO A RELATIONSHIP, AND, ACCORDING TO THIS THEORY, A COUPLE IS WELL-MATCHED IF THEIR TRIANGLES LOOK ALIKE.

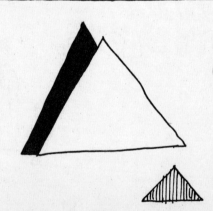

MOMMY! DADDY! JUSTIN CALLED ME A SQUARE!

STERNBERG ISN'T THE ONLY ONE TRYING TO DISSECT LOVE. SEVERAL OTHER PSYCHOLOGISTS HAVE SOUGHT THE LOVE OF THEIR PEERS BY CREATING THEORIES OF LOVE.

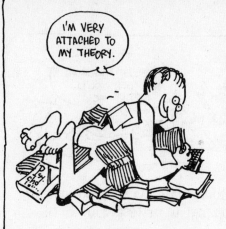

I'M VERY ATTACHED TO MY THEORY.

ATTACHMENT THEORY ANALYZES THE ABILITY TO FORM LOVING ATTACHMENTS IN TERMS OF THE RELATIONSHIP WITH THE EARLIEST CAREGIVER (USUALLY A PERSON'S MOTHER). IF THIS RELATIONSHIP WAS "SECURE," THEN ADULT RELATIONSHIPS ARE SUPPOSED TO BE COMFORTABLE, AND THE PERSON SHOULD BE TRUSTING, HAPPY, AND SUPPORTIVE. IF YOU HAVE PROBLEMS WITH INTIMACY AND LOVE, ATTACHMENT THEORY WOULD TEND TO BLAME YOUR MOM!

SOCIOLOGIST **JOHN LEE** CLASSIFIES LOVE ACCORDING TO STYLE. THERE ARE SIX STYLES:

1.) LOVE OF BEAUTY: ROMANTIC, PASSIONATE, AND FLEETING
2.) OBSESSIVE LOVE
3.) PLAYFUL LOVE: "NOTHING SERIOUS"
4.) COMPANIONATE OR FRIENDLY LOVE
5.) PRACTICAL, RATIONAL LOVE
6.) SELF-SACRIFICING LOVE

LEE ADORNS EACH STYLE WITH A SCIENTIFIC-SOUNDING GRECO-LATIN NAME, WHICH WE FORGET AT THE MOMENT.

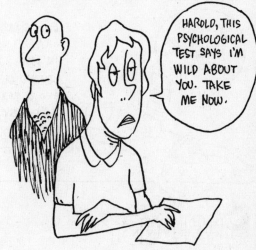

HAROLD, THIS PSYCHOLOGICAL TEST SAYS I'M WILD ABOUT YOU. TAKE ME NOW.

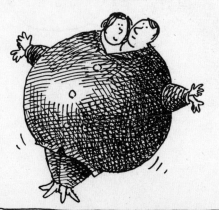

SOCIAL PSYCHOLOGISTS **ART & ELAINE ARON** SEE LOVERS AS DRIVEN BY A DESIRE TO EXPAND THEIR OWN INDIVIDUAL PERSPECTIVES, RESOURCES, AND IDENTITIES.

LOVE PROBLEMS

LOVE ISN'T ALWAYS A SOURCE OF JOY. SOMETIMES IT CAN MAKE US MISERABLE...

UNREQUITED LOVE

CAN DRIVE PEOPLE NUTS... WHY WOULD ANYONE PERSIST IN PURSUING A LOVE INTEREST WHO DOESN'T RETURN THE FEELING?

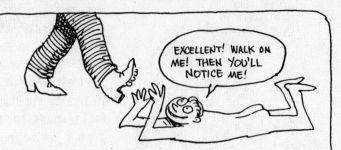

EXCELLENT! WALK ON ME! THEN YOU'LL NOTICE ME!

ATTACHMENT THEORISTS WOULD SAY THAT THE UNREQUITED LOVER HAS A POOR ATTACHMENT STYLE. A MORE SECURE PERSON, SAYS THE THEORY, WOULD GIVE UP THE OBSESSION AND FIND SOMEONE MORE CARING AND SATISFYING.

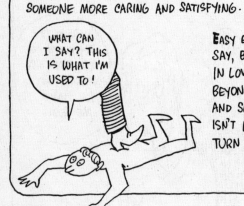

WHAT CAN I SAY? THIS IS WHAT I'M USED TO!

EASY ENOUGH TO SAY, BUT WE FALL IN LOVE FOR REASONS BEYOND OUR CONTROL, AND SOMETIMES IT ISN'T EASY TO TURN IT OFF!

I'LL COMPROMISE. I'LL SLEEP WITH YOU AND THINK OF HIM!

UM... THANKS... I GUESS...

JEALOUSY

IS ANOTHER LOVE-HORROR. SOMETIMES THE JEALOUS LOVER IS IRRATIONALLY SUSPICIOUS... AT OTHER TIMES, RATIONALLY SUSPICIOUS... AT STILL OTHER TIMES, THE LOVER IS REACTING TO SOMETHING THAT HAS ALREADY HAPPENED. JEALOUSY CAN BE SEXUAL OR PURELY EMOTIONAL, AS WHEN A PARTNER APPEARS TO CARE TOO MUCH FOR SOMEONE ELSE.

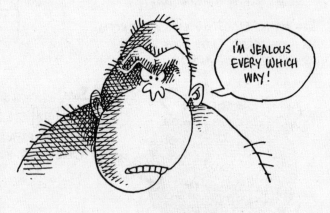

I'M JEALOUS EVERY WHICH WAY!

SOMETIMES, A LOVER CAN RISE ABOVE JEALOUSY, AND THE THREE PARTIES CAN WORK THINGS OUT WITH A MINIMUM OF BAD CONSEQUENCES.

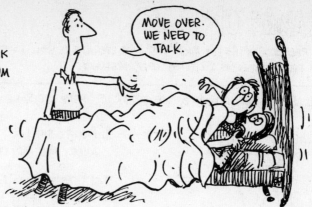

AT OTHER TIMES, JEALOUSY BRINGS ON A CRISIS IN A RELATIONSHIP THAT CAN'T BE RESOLVED.

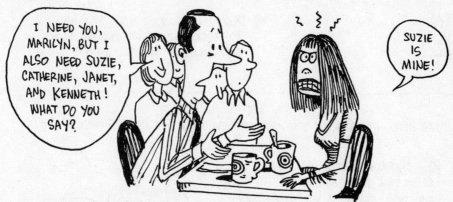

AND EVERY NOW AND THEN, JEALOUSY FLARES UP INTO AN UNCONTROLLABLE FURY THAT LEADS TO VIOLENCE AND DEATH...

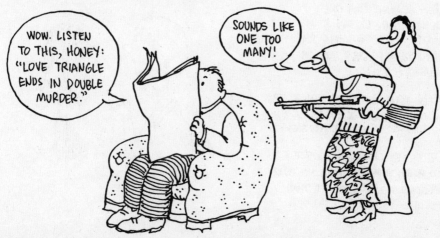

BREAKING UP

IF THE RELATIONSHIP REALLY MUST END (AND EVERYONE IS STILL ALIVE!), THE ETIQUETTE ELF HAS A FEW POINTERS ON SPLITTING UP GRACEFULLY:

IF YOU ARE THE ONE INITIATING THE BREAK-UP, HERE ARE SOME RULES:

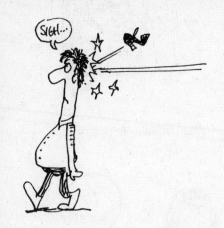

1. ACCEPT THE FACT THAT YOUR MATE WILL BE ANGRY AND MAY CAST YOU AS THE VILLAIN.

2. IF POSSIBLE, DON'T LIE TO SPARE YOUR MATE'S FEELINGS. WHEN THE TRUTH DOES COME OUT, YOUR EX-TO-BE WILL BE TWICE AS MAD!

3. SEEING YOUR FORMER MATE AFTERWARDS "AS FRIENDS" IS USUALLY A BAD IDEA.

4. DON'T CHANGE YOUR MIND JUST BECAUSE YOU FEEL LONELY. THE REASONS BEHIND THE BREAK-UP ARE STILL THERE.

ON THE OTHER HAND, IF YOU'RE ON THE RECEIVING END OF A BREAK-UP, REMEMBER —

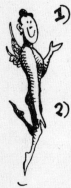

1) PAIN AND LONELINESS AND ANGER ARE NATURAL CONSEQUENCES OF REJECTION. THEY ARE NOT NECESSARILY A SIGN THAT YOU ARE STILL IN LOVE! YOU **WILL** GET OVER IT.

2) JUST BECAUSE THIS ONE DUMPED YOU, YOU ARE STILL WORTHY OF LOVE. SPEND TIME WITH YOUR FRIENDS, AND TREAT YOURSELF WELL.

3) KEEP YOUR SENSE OF HUMOR. TRY IMAGINING YOUR EX SPEAKING NAKED TO THE REPUBLICAN CONVENTION.

4) DO NOT STALK, HARASS, OR TRY TO HARM YOUR EX. FEELING BAD AT HOME IS MUCH BETTER THAN FEELING BAD IN JAIL!!

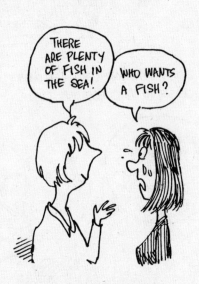

STAYING TOGETHER

And if we don't break up? What then? Is it possible to sustain romance, passion, and love through years of daily exposure, disagreements, negotiations, children, and physical decay? Could be!

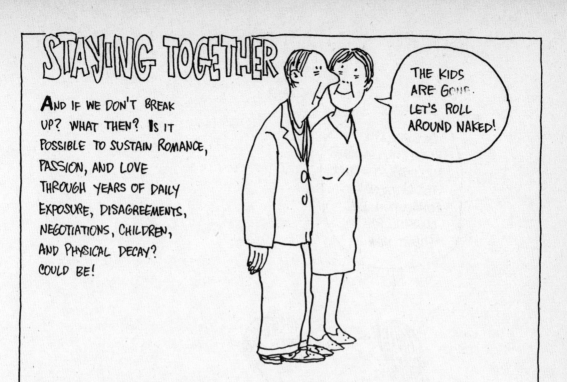

Although passion usually fades, it may not disappear entirely... and if we do the work necessary to make a shared life with someone, we can have the comfort, the satisfaction, and, yes, the thrill of knowing that someone still wants us after 20, 30, or 50 years. That's love, too — and that's not bad!!

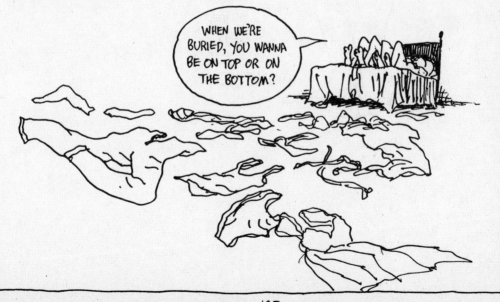

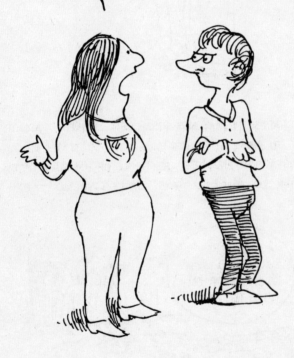

·· CHAPTER 8 ··

IT, AS IN "DOING IT"
(OR, AS THE EXPERTS CALL IT, SEXUAL EXPRESSION)

So far, this book has circled around its subject like a nervous male pigeon courting his mate. We've looked at sex in nature, sex as a part of growing up, and sex as a part of identity. We've communicated about sex and fallen in love... but what about the prize at the center of it all? What about the sex act itself, or, to be more precise, sex acts, since people express their sexual urges in many different ways?

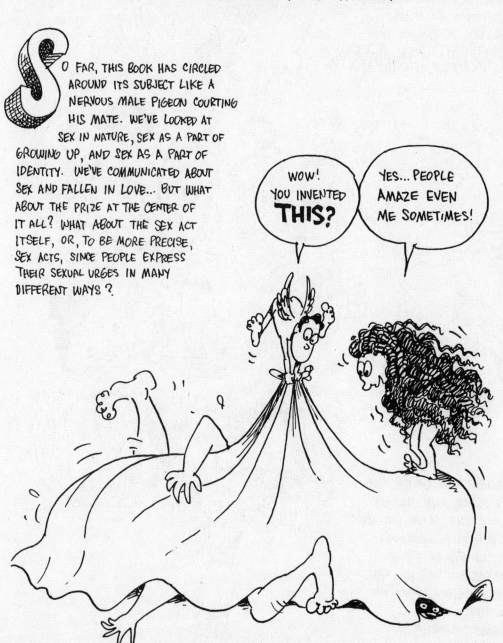

WOW! YOU INVENTED **THIS?**

YES... PEOPLE AMAZE EVEN ME SOMETIMES!

FREUD WOULD SAY OUR FIRST EROTIC EXPERIENCE COMES AT OUR MOTHER'S BREAST, BUT SINCE WE CAN'T INTERVIEW BABIES, LET'S FAST-FORWARD TO A FORM OF SEXUAL EXPRESSION MOST OF US DEFINITELY DO ENGAGE IN: SEXUAL FANTASY.

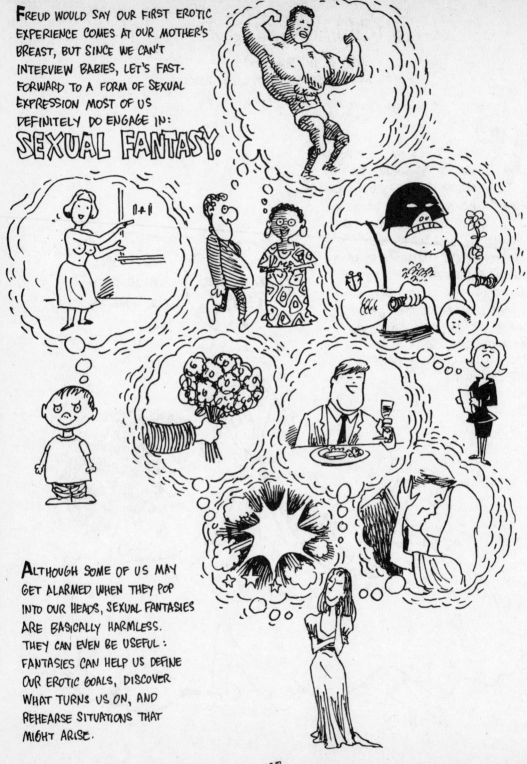

ALTHOUGH SOME OF US MAY GET ALARMED WHEN THEY POP INTO OUR HEADS, SEXUAL FANTASIES ARE BASICALLY HARMLESS. THEY CAN EVEN BE USEFUL: FANTASIES CAN HELP US DEFINE OUR EROTIC GOALS, DISCOVER WHAT TURNS US ON, AND REHEARSE SITUATIONS THAT MIGHT ARISE.

128

FANTASIES MAY BE JOINED BY ANOTHER
SOLITARY FORM OF SEXUAL EXPRESSION:

MASTURBATION.

MOST KIDS FIGURE OUT PRETTY EARLY
THAT IT FEELS GOOD DOWN THERE.

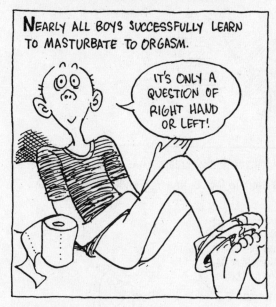

NEARLY ALL BOYS SUCCESSFULLY LEARN
TO MASTURBATE TO ORGASM.

IT'S ONLY A QUESTION OF RIGHT HAND OR LEFT!

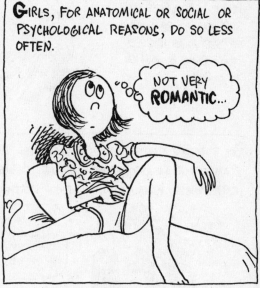

GIRLS, FOR ANATOMICAL OR SOCIAL OR
PSYCHOLOGICAL REASONS, DO SO LESS
OFTEN.

NOT VERY ROMANTIC...

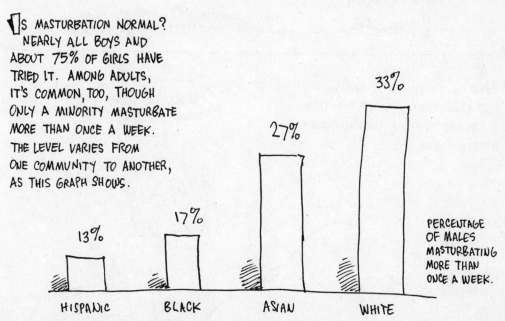

IS MASTURBATION NORMAL?
NEARLY ALL BOYS AND
ABOUT 75% OF GIRLS HAVE
TRIED IT. AMONG ADULTS,
IT'S COMMON, TOO, THOUGH
ONLY A MINORITY MASTURBATE
MORE THAN ONCE A WEEK.
THE LEVEL VARIES FROM
ONE COMMUNITY TO ANOTHER,
AS THIS GRAPH SHOWS.

33%

27%

17%

13%

HISPANIC

BLACK

ASIAN

WHITE

PERCENTAGE
OF MALES
MASTURBATING
MORE THAN
ONCE A WEEK.

THE JUDAEO-CHRISTIAN
TRADITION HAS ALWAYS
FROWNED ON MASTURBATION,
AT LEAST FOR BOYS. (THE
TRADITION NEVER NOTICED OR
ADMITTED THAT GIRLS
DO IT!) FOR BOYS, IT'S
SUPPOSED TO BE A WASTE
OF "SEED," AS IF SEED
DIDN'T COME 60 MILLION
TO A POP.

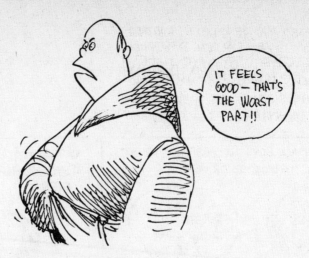

IT FEELS
GOOD — THAT'S
THE WORST
PART!!

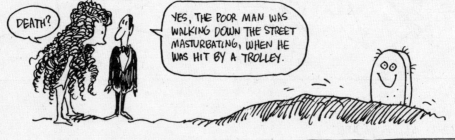

BY THE 19TH CENTURY THIS DISAPPROVAL HAD BEEN MEDICALIZED. MASTURBATION WAS
BLAMED FOR AN ASSORTMENT OF ILLS: IT WAS SAID TO CAUSE HAIRY HANDS, WARTS,
NERVOUSNESS, EXHAUSTION, AND EVEN DEATH.

DEATH?

YES, THE POOR MAN WAS
WALKING DOWN THE STREET
MASTURBATING, WHEN HE
WAS HIT BY A TROLLEY.

NOW THAT EVERYONE IS NERVOUS
AND EXHAUSTED MOST OF THE TIME,
ATTITUDES TOWARDS MASTURBATION
HAVE CHANGED.

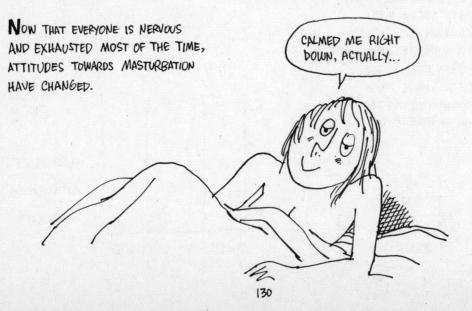

CALMED ME RIGHT
DOWN, ACTUALLY...

EVENTUALLY, THOUGH, MOST OF US WOULD LIKE TO EXPRESS OURSELVES SEXUALLY WITH SOMEONE ELSE. WHAT THEN? THE FIRST THING WOULD BE TO FIND THAT PERSON AND SHARE ALL THE PRELIMINARY COMMUNICATION OF CHAPTER 6... UNTIL THE TWO OF YOU "GET TO YES."

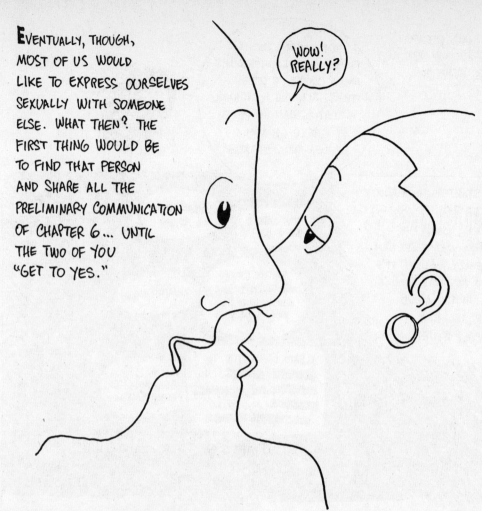

O.K.! NOW YOU'RE IN THE MOOD... OOPS! DON'T FORGET TO HAVE **THE CONVERSATION!!**

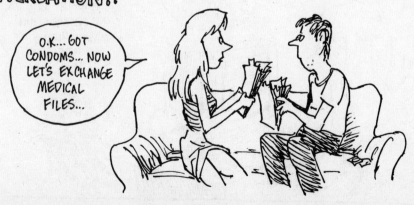

O.K... THAT'S OUT OF THE WAY, AND NOW YOU'RE READY TO... WHAT?

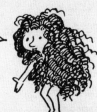

NOTE: EXCEPT FOR PENILE-VAGINAL INTERCOURSE AND A COUPLE OF OTHER ITEMS, ALL THE FOLLOWING ACTIVITIES CAN BE DONE BY PEOPLE OF ANY GENDER AND ORIENTATION!

FOR STARTERS, HOW ABOUT **TALKING?** TALKING ABOUT SEX CAN BE REALLY... SEXY! IT'S NOT A BAD WAY TO GET BACK IN THE MOOD AFTER ALL THAT DIFFICULT STUFF...

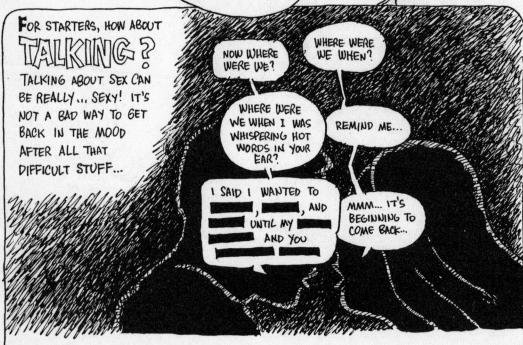

IF YOU NEED ANY PROOF THAT TALK CAN BE SEXY, JUST LOOK AT HOW POPULAR PHONE SEX IS... OR INTERNET SEX CHAT.

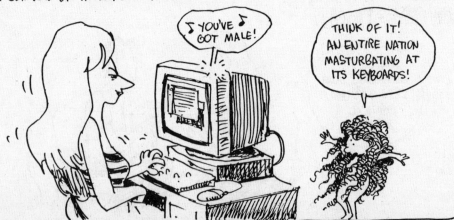

NEXT WOULD COME **KISSING.** DURING ADOLESCENCE, LEARNING TO KISS WELL IS A NEAR OBSESSION.

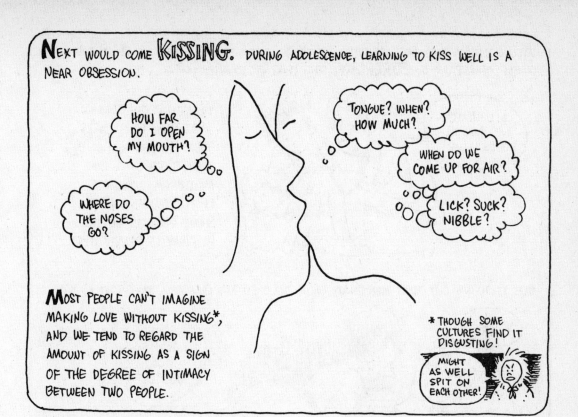

MOST PEOPLE CAN'T IMAGINE MAKING LOVE WITHOUT KISSING*, AND WE TEND TO REGARD THE AMOUNT OF KISSING AS A SIGN OF THE DEGREE OF INTIMACY BETWEEN TWO PEOPLE.

KISSES COME IN ALL KINDS:

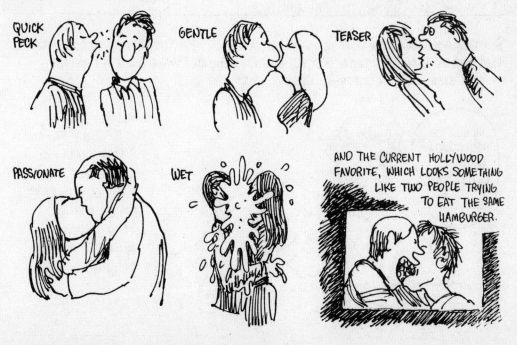

ALONG WITH KISSING GOES TOUCHING... PETTING... "MAKING OUT"... THIS CAN BE AN END IN ITSELF OR A PART OF **FOREPLAY,** THE LEAD-UP TO INTERCOURSE.

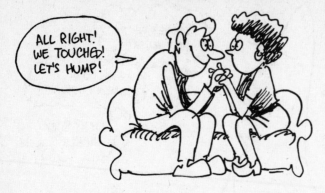

ALL RIGHT! WE TOUCHED! LET'S HUMP!

WOMEN OFTEN COMPLAIN THAT MEN DON'T CARESS THEM ENOUGH TO REALLY TURN THEM ON... THAT MEN SEEM TO VIEW A LITTLE TOUCHING AS A SHORT ON-RAMP TO THE HIGHWAY OF PENETRATION...

BUT IT TURNS OUT THAT MEN ENJOY BEING TOUCHED AND CARESSED, TOO... WHAT A SURPRISE!

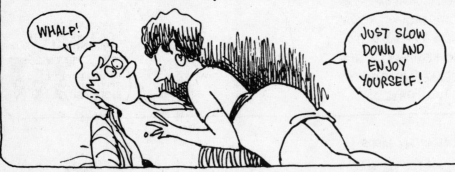

WHALP!

JUST SLOW DOWN AND ENJOY YOURSELF!

SEX THERAPISTS MAY RECOMMEND THIS EXERCISE TO COUPLES: PARTNERS TAKE TURNS EXPLORING EACH OTHERS' BODIES, TOUCHING ANYTHING BUT THE GENITALS, WHILE THE OTHER PARTNER REPORTS BACK HOW IT ALL FEELS. ORGASM IS NOT THE GOAL!

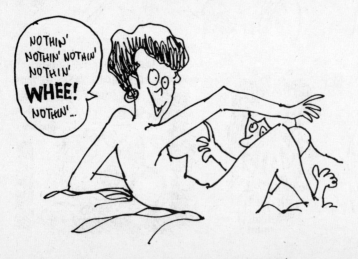

NOTHIN' NOTHIN' NOTHIN' NOTHIN' **WHEE!** NOTHIN'...

THIS MAY SEEM A LITTLE TOO SYSTEMATIC OR COLD-BLOODED TO SOME PEOPLE, BUT IT IS UNQUESTIONABLY A GOOD WAY TO LEARN SOMETHING ABOUT A PARTNER'S RESPONSES.

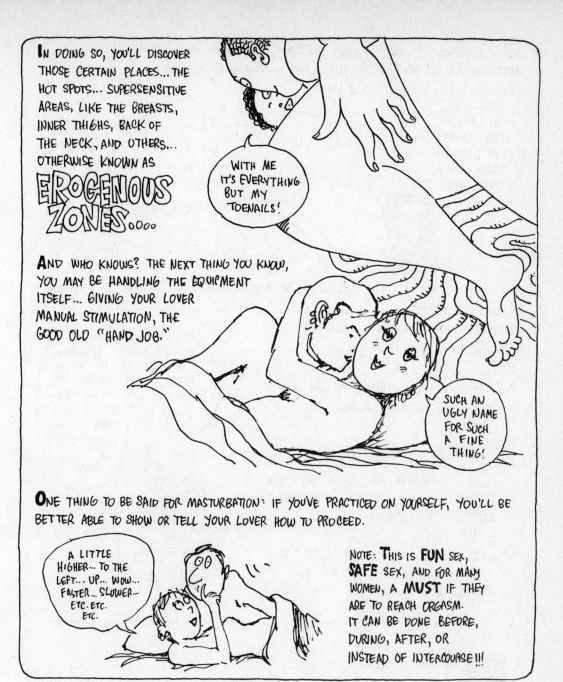

IN DOING SO, YOU'LL DISCOVER THOSE CERTAIN PLACES... THE HOT SPOTS... SUPERSENSITIVE AREAS, LIKE THE BREASTS, INNER THIGHS, BACK OF THE NECK, AND OTHERS... OTHERWISE KNOWN AS

EROGENOUS ZONES....

WITH ME IT'S EVERYTHING BUT MY TOENAILS!

AND WHO KNOWS? THE NEXT THING YOU KNOW, YOU MAY BE HANDLING THE EQUIPMENT ITSELF... GIVING YOUR LOVER MANUAL STIMULATION, THE GOOD OLD "HAND JOB."

SUCH AN UGLY NAME FOR SUCH A FINE THING!

ONE THING TO BE SAID FOR MASTURBATION: IF YOU'VE PRACTICED ON YOURSELF, YOU'LL BE BETTER ABLE TO SHOW OR TELL YOUR LOVER HOW TO PROCEED.

A LITTLE HIGHER... TO THE LEFT... UP... WOW... FASTER... SLOWER... ETC. ETC. ETC.

NOTE: THIS IS **FUN** SEX, **SAFE** SEX, AND FOR MANY WOMEN, A **MUST** IF THEY ARE TO REACH ORGASM. IT CAN BE DONE BEFORE, DURING, AFTER, OR INSTEAD OF INTERCOURSE!!!

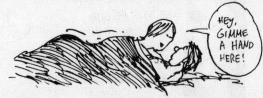

HEY, GIMME A HAND HERE!

WITH KISSING, LIP-TO-LIP IS ONLY THE BEGINNING. NIBBLING, LICKING, SUCKING, AND BITING (BUT GENTLY!) CAN HAPPEN ANYWHERE: FINGERS, TOES, NIPPLES... YOU NAME IT!

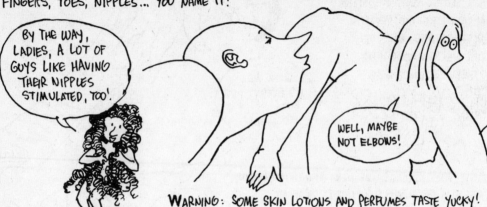

BY THE WAY, LADIES, A LOT OF GUYS LIKE HAVING THEIR NIPPLES STIMULATED, TOO!

WELL, MAYBE NOT ELBOWS!

WARNING: SOME SKIN LOTIONS AND PERFUMES TASTE YUCKY!

HEADING SOUTH, WE ENTER THE REALM OF

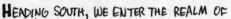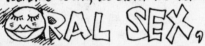 **ORAL SEX,**

THE STIMULATION OF GENITALS BY LIPS AND TONGUE. THIS COMES IN TWO BASIC FLAVORS — ER, VERSIONS.

WHY DO THERE HAVE TO BE ALL THESE LATIN WORDS?

IT WOULD BE ÷AHEM÷ INDELICATE TO SAY "BLOW JOB" OR "GIVE HEAD" OR "MUFF DIVE" OR "GO DOWN"...

◆ **CUNNILINGUS:** (FROM LATIN "CUNNI-", THE VULVA, AND "LINGUS", THE TONGUE). KISSING OR LICKING THE FEMALE SEX ORGANS, ESPECIALLY THE CLITORIS.

◆ **FELLATIO:** (FROM LATIN "FELLARE," TO SUCK) PRETENDING THE PENIS IS A POPSICLE.

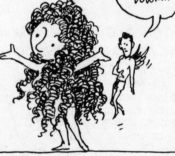

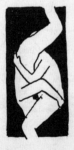 THESE CAN BE DONE ONE AT A TIME OR TWO AT ONCE, IN THE POSITION KNOWN IN FRENCH AS "SOIXANTE-NEUF" (SIXTY-NINE).

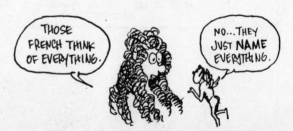

THOSE FRENCH THINK OF EVERYTHING.

NO...THEY JUST **NAME** EVERYTHING.

136

WOMEN ARE OF TWO MINDS ABOUT CUNNILINGUS. NEARLY ALL OF THEM AGREE IT FEELS GOOD...

BUT THEY WORRY THAT THEIR PARTNER MAY FIND THE ACT DISTASTEFUL.

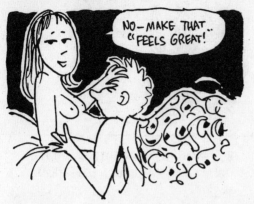

NO—MAKE THAT.. "FEELS GREAT!

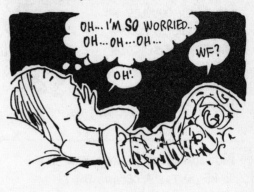

OH... I'M SO WORRIED.. OH...OH...OH...

OH'.

WF?

IN FACT, A LARGE MAJORITY OF MEN (AROUND 75%) SAY THEY LIKE PERFORMING CUNNILINGUS.

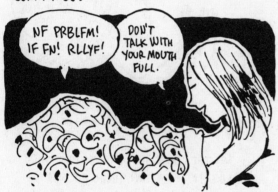

NF PRBLFM! IF FN! RLLYF!

DON'T TALK WITH YOUR MOUTH FULL.

THE REASON, THEY SAY, IS THAT THEY LIKE TURNING THEIR PARTNER ON... AND THEY THINK SHE TASTES JUST FINE!! (IF SHE DOESN'T, IT MAY BE A SYMPTOM OF A VAGINAL INFECTION.)

AMONG LESBIAN COUPLES, A SURVEY FOUND SATISFACTION AND HAPPINESS TO BE HIGHER IN THOSE COUPLES THAT PRACTICED CUNNILINGUS THAN IN THOSE THAT DID NOT.

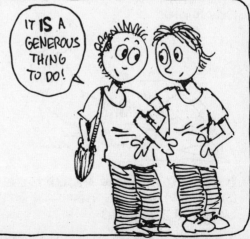

IT IS A GENEROUS THING TO DO!

LIKEWISE, AMONG GAY MEN, FELLATIO IS THE PREFERRED SEX ACT, AND AGAIN COUPLES WHO DO IT TEND TO REPORT GREATER SATISFACTION THAN COUPLES WHO DON'T.

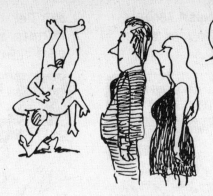

NOW THERE GOES A HAPPY COUPLE!

NOT SURPRISINGLY, MOST MEN LIKE TO BE ON THE RECEIVING END OF ORAL SEX...

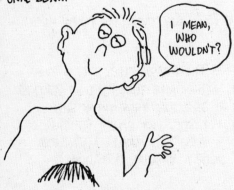

I MEAN, WHO WOULDN'T?

ABOUT HALF OF ALL WOMEN WON'T DO IT AT ALL. SOME WHO DO RESENT IT AS A KIND OF SUBMISSION — ESPECIALLY IF THEIR PARTNER DOESN'T REPAY THE FAVOR IN KIND.

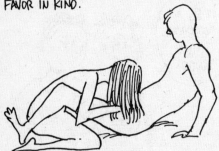

IT MAY ALSO BE HARDER FOR A WOMAN TO KEEP CONTROL WHEN PERFORMING FELLATIO. SHE RISKS GAGGING OR BEING FORCED.

BUT MANY WOMEN'S ENTHUSIASM FOR FELLATIO IS DECIDEDLY LESS THAN HIGH...

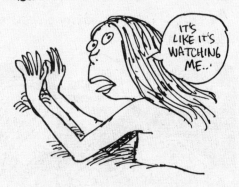

IT'S LIKE IT'S WATCHING ME...

ON THE OTHER HAND, MANY WOMEN DO LIKE IT. EXCITING THEIR PARTNER EXCITES THEM... AND BESIDES, THERE'S SOMETHING NASTY AND THRILLING ABOUT THE ACT...

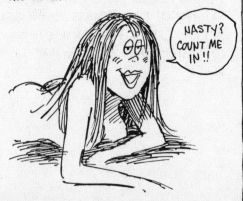

NASTY? COUNT ME IN!!

FINALLY, THERE'S THE AGE-OLD QUESTION: TO SWALLOW OR NOT TO SWALLOW?

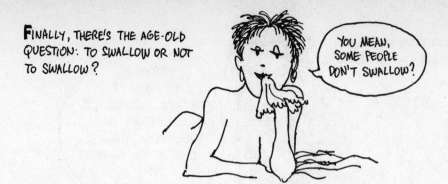

YOU MEAN, SOME PEOPLE DON'T SWALLOW?

SOME WOMEN DON'T LIKE THE IDEA OF SEMEN IN THEIR MOUTH, OR AT LEAST NOT IN THEIR STOMACH. THIS RAISES SOME DELICATE ISSUES OF ETIQUETTE. HERE ARE SOME POINTERS.

GUYS, DON'T TAKE IT PERSONALLY IF YOUR PARTNER WON'T LET YOU COME IN HER OR HIS MOUTH. THIS PERSON HAS DONE A NICE THING FOR YOU. BE GRATEFUL!

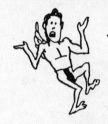

IF YOU DON'T SWALLOW, BE GRACIOUS! DON'T JUST LET THAT PENIS FLAIL AROUND ON ITS OWN. BE NICE TO ITS OWNER!

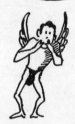

IF POSSIBLE, DON'T GAG, RETCH, OR ACT AS IF YOU'RE HAVING A BAD TIME. IF THE ACT IS UNPLEASANT, DON'T DO IT!

HEALTH NOTE: ORAL SEX, ESPECIALLY FELLATIO, IS NOT RISK-FREE. SEMEN CAN CARRY H.I.V. OR OTHER STDs... SEX ORGANS CAN HAVE HERPES LESIONS OR WARTS THAT MAY BE TRANSMITTED TO LIPS OR MOUTH... SO, UNLESS YOU'RE ABSOLUTELY SURE YOUR PARTNER IS HIV-FREE (AND FAIRLY SURE ABOUT OTHER STDs), YOU SHOULD AVOID ORAL SEX, UNLESS YOU CAN GET USED TO USING A CONDOM.

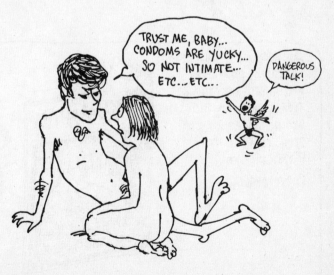

TRUST ME, BABY... CONDOMS ARE YUCKY... SO NOT INTIMATE... ETC...ETC...

DANGEROUS TALK!

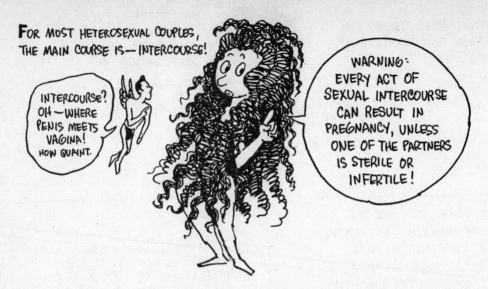

FOR MOST HETEROSEXUAL COUPLES, THE MAIN COURSE IS—INTERCOURSE!

INTERCOURSE? OH—WHERE PENIS MEETS VAGINA! HOW QUANT.

WARNING: EVERY ACT OF SEXUAL INTERCOURSE CAN RESULT IN PREGNANCY, UNLESS ONE OF THE PARTNERS IS STERILE OR INFERTILE!

THROUGHOUT HISTORY, PEOPLE HAVE LOOKED FOR NEW WAYS TO DO IT, WAYS TO MAKE IT LAST LONGER, WAYS TO PUMP UP THE EXCITEMENT, ETC.,ETC., ETC. WE ARE AN IMAGINATIVE AND EXPERIMENTAL SPECIES!

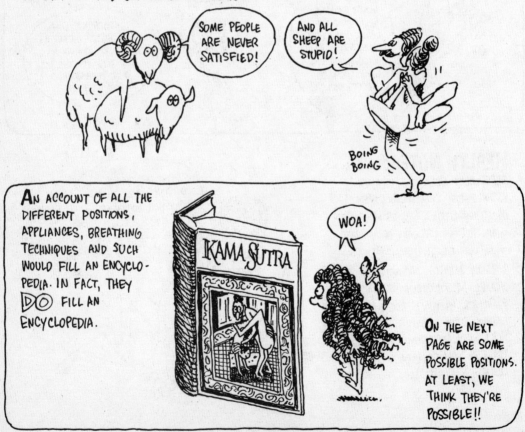

SOME PEOPLE ARE NEVER SATISFIED!

AND ALL SHEEP ARE STUPID!

BOING BOING

AN ACCOUNT OF ALL THE DIFFERENT POSITIONS, APPLIANCES, BREATHING TECHNIQUES AND SUCH WOULD FILL AN ENCYCLOPEDIA. IN FACT, THEY DO FILL AN ENCYCLOPEDIA.

KAMA SUTRA

WOA!

ON THE NEXT PAGE ARE SOME POSSIBLE POSITIONS. AT LEAST, WE THINK THEY'RE POSSIBLE!!

MALE ABOVE

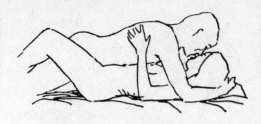

FEMALE ABOVE

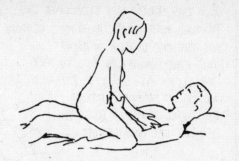

ON SIDE, FACE TO FACE

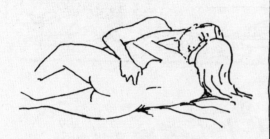

ON SIDE, BACK TO FRONT

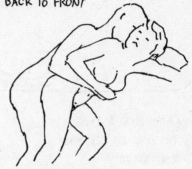

SITTING

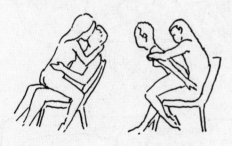

STANDING (NOT FOR PEOPLE WITH BAD KNEES!)

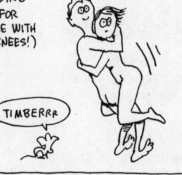

TIMBERRR

ON FURNITURE

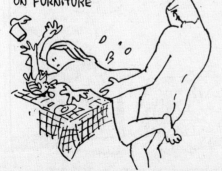

ETC.!

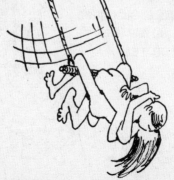

141

ALL THIS ACTION MAY STIMULATE ONE PARTNER MORE THAN THE OTHER. USUALLY HE'S THE ONE CLOSER TO CLIMAX. IN THIS CASE, IT MAY BE TIME TO HELP HER ALONG WITH A LITTLE EXTRA ATTENTION TO THE CLITORIS — AND HOLD HIMSELF BACK WITH SOME MENTAL GYMNASTICS.

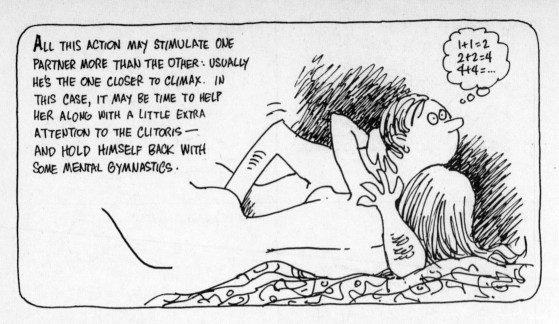

$$1+1=2$$
$$2+2=4$$
$$4+4=\dots$$

ONCE UPON A TIME, THE GOAL OF SEX WAS SUPPOSED TO BE

SIMULTANEOUS ORGASM.

IF BOTH PARTNERS DIDN'T "COME TOGETHER," SOMEBODY WAS OUT OF LUCK.

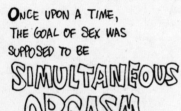

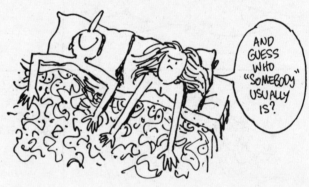

AND GUESS WHO "SOMEBODY" USUALLY IS?

NOW, IN AN ERA OF MUTUALITY AND COMMUNICATION, THERE IS NO REASON WHY BOTH PARTNERS CAN'T HAVE AN ORGASM, IN WHATEVER ORDER THEY DECIDE.

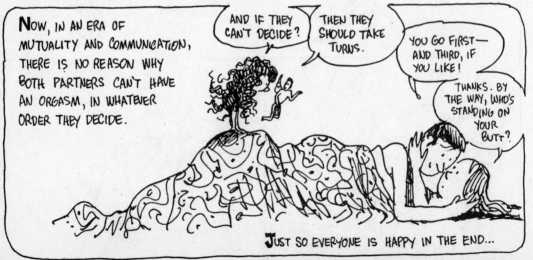

AND IF THEY CAN'T DECIDE?

THEN THEY SHOULD TAKE TURNS.

YOU GO FIRST— AND THIRD, IF YOU LIKE!

THANKS. BY THE WAY, WHO'S STANDING ON YOUR BUTT?

JUST SO EVERYONE IS HAPPY IN THE END...

AND SPEAKING OF THE END...

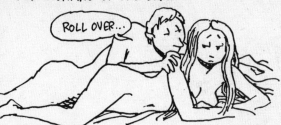

ROLL OVER...

MANY PEOPLE FIND ANAL STIMULATION AROUSING. THIS INCLUDES CARESSING WITH THE FINGERS, LICKING ("ANALINGUS"), AND PENETRATION BY FINGERS OR PENIS.

ABOUT ¼ OF HETERO ADULTS HAVE TRIED ANAL INTERCOURSE. FOR MOST OF THEM, IT APPEARS TO BE AN EXPERIMENTAL ACTIVITY.

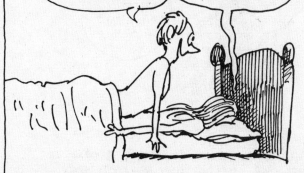

OH, DARLENE, THAT WAS A ONCE-IN-A-LIFETIME EXPERIENCE!

YUP IT WAS, IF I HAVE ANYTHING TO SAY ABOUT IT...

ON THE OTHER HAND, SOME COUPLES DO IT REGULARLY.

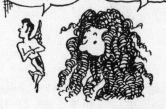

IT'S ONE WAY NOT TO GET PREGNANT!

AND NOT UNCOMMON AMONG GAY MEN.

BUT — THERE HAD TO BE A "BUT" HERE, DIDN'T THERE? HERE'S A BIG

HEALTH WARNING:

ANAL SEX IS **RISKY!** RECTAL TISSUE IS EASILY DAMAGED, ALLOWING VIRUSES LIKE HIV TO ENTER THE BLOODSTREAM. ANAL PENETRATION IS A GREAT SPREADER OF AIDS.

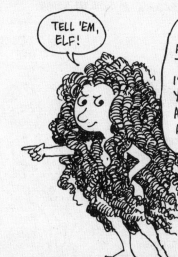

TELL 'EM, ELF!

IF YOU ARE NOT ABSOLUTELY SURE THAT YOUR PARTNER IS FREE OF H.I.V., YOU **MUST** USE A CONDOM DURING ANAL AND VAGINAL INTERCOURSE!

NO IFS, ANDS, OR... OH, NEVER MIND...

SINCE SOME 25% OF COUPLES HAVE AT LEAST TRIED ANAL SEX, IT IS CONSIDERED NORMAL BEHAVIOR (IN SENSE #2. SEE P. 72.) OTHER, LESS COMMON ACTIVITIES ARE CALLED

atypical

BEHAVIORS.

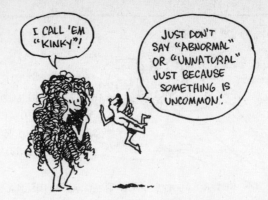

I CALL 'EM "KINKY"!

JUST DON'T SAY "ABNORMAL" OR "UNNATURAL" JUST BECAUSE SOMETHING IS UNCOMMON!

AND BEYOND THE FRINGE OF THE FRINGE ARE BEHAVIORS THAT ARE CONSIDERED ILLNESSES, SYMPTOMS OF MENTAL DISTURBANCE. THERE'S A NAME FOR THESE TOO, AND OF COURSE IT COMES FROM THE GREEK:

PARAPHiLiA

(MEANING LOVE OF THE IRREGULAR).

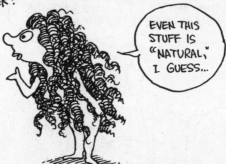

EVEN THIS STUFF IS "NATURAL," I GUESS...

THE LINE BETWEEN ATYPICAL BEHAVIOR AND PARAPHILIA IS NOT ALWAYS EASY TO DRAW. TO SOME EXTENT, IT'S IN THE EYE OF THE BEHOLDER... AND DIFFERENT BEHOLDERS HAVE DIFFERENT EYES. ONCE UPON A TIME, NOT MUCH OF ANYTHING WAS TOLERATED, ASIDE FROM MAN-ON-TOP INTERCOURSE WITHIN MARRIAGE.

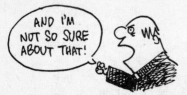

AND I'M NOT SO SURE ABOUT THAT!

WELL, THERE'S A RELIEF!

AS LONG AS YOU'RE HAPPY...

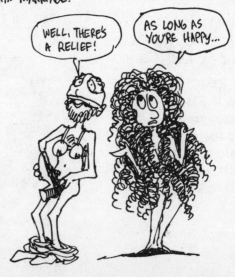

A LESS JUDGMENTAL VIEW IS THIS: PARAPHILIAS ARE CHARACTERIZED BY RECURRENT, INTENSE FANTASIES OR URGES. THEY MAY INVOLVE CHILDREN OR OTHER NON-CONSENTING PEOPLE... OR REAL (NOT SIMULATED) SUFFERING AND HUMILIATION... AND FINALLY, THE URGES AND BEHAVIORS MAY BE DISTRESSING TO THE PERSON WHO HAS OR DOES THEM.

ANOTHER EXAMPLE OF ATYPICAL
SEXUAL BEHAVIOR — AROUND
10% OF MEN AND WOMEN
HAVE TRIED IT — IS
PLAYING OUT ROLES OF
DOMINANCE AND
SUBMISSION... (D/S)

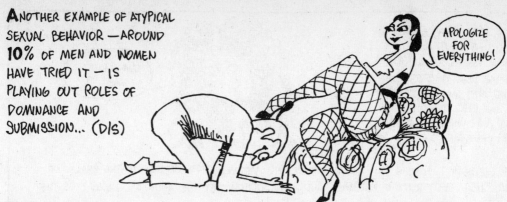

APOLOGIZE
FOR
EVERYTHING!

THERE'S NO DENYING THAT POWER HAS A SEXUAL CHARGE... AND SOME COUPLES
GET OFF BY ACTING OUT SCENES IN WHICH ONE PERSON DOMINATES AND THE OTHER
SUBMITS (SOMETIMES PRETENDING TO RESIST). THESE GAMES NEED GROUND RULES!

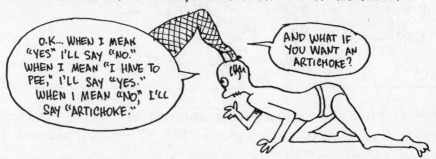

O.K... WHEN I MEAN
"YES" I'LL SAY "NO."
WHEN I MEAN "I HAVE TO
PEE," I'LL SAY "YES."
WHEN I MEAN "NO," I'LL
SAY "ARTICHOKE."

AND WHAT IF
YOU WANT AN
ARTICHOKE?

THE MOST WIDELY-KNOWN FORM OF D/S IS BONDAGE AND DISCIPLINE, OR B&D.
B&D INVOLVES SIMULATED OR LIGHT DISCIPLINARY ACTIVITIES, SUCH AS SPANKING,
PERFORMED ON A PARTNER WHO IS RESTRAINED BY SCARVES, STRAPS, ROPES,
HANDCUFFS, ETC., ETC., ETC...

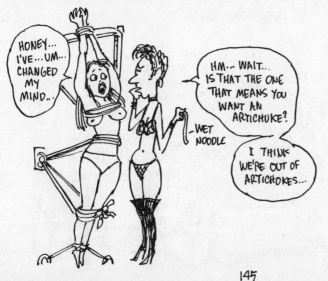

HONEY...
I'VE...UM...
CHANGED
MY
MIND...

HM... WAIT...
IS THAT THE ONE
THAT MEANS YOU
WANT AN
ARTICHOKE?

— WET
NOODLE

I THINK
WE'RE OUT OF
ARTICHOKES...

WARNING!
THIS GAME IS ONLY
FOR PEOPLE WHO TRUST
EACH OTHER, AND IT'S
ONLY O.K. IF BOTH
PARTNERS ARE WILLING!!

As long as it's all fun and games, B&D is harmless enough... but where does it cross the line into sadism (delight in the infliction of pain) and masochism (the need to feel pain)?

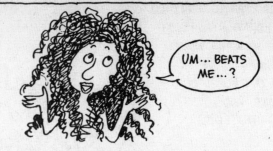

UM... BEATS ME...?

If the sadist forces pain on an unwilling victim, we're clearly in the realm of paraphilia. But what if a sadist and a masochist get together willingly? Is that paraphilia??

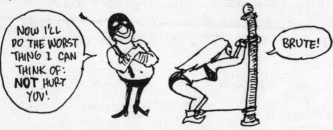

NOW I'LL DO THE WORST THING I CAN THINK OF: **NOT** HURT YOU!

BRUTE!

Another example is cross-dressing, or transvestism. Most transvestites get off by wearing the clothes of the other sex — almost always a man wearing women's clothing.

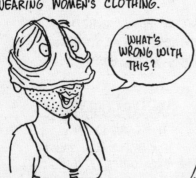

WHAT'S WRONG WITH THIS?

Psychologists usually consider transvestism to be a paraphilia, at least when it's done furtively and compulsively by heterosexual men who feel weird about it...

But among gay men, it's much much more open... and people cross-dress for other reasons besides sexual thrills: as a parody of gender roles, as a way of declaring a sexual identity (for gays and lesbians), or for "gender comfort."

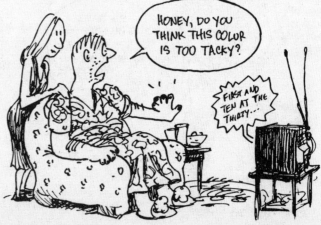

HONEY, DO YOU THINK THIS COLOR IS TOO TACKY?

FIRST AND TEN AT THE THIRTY...

FOR ANOTHER EXAMPLE: MASTURBATION IS NORMAL... FREQUENT MASTURBATION IS ATYPICAL... AND COMPULSIVE MASTURBATION, WHICH MEANS FREQUENT, REGULAR MASTURBATION TO THE EXCLUSION OF OTHER SEXUAL ACTIVITY, WOULD BE CONSIDERED A PARAPHILIA.

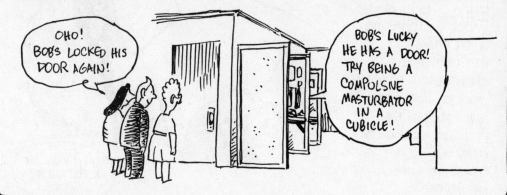

OHO! BOB'S LOCKED HIS DOOR AGAIN!

BOB'S LUCKY HE HAS A DOOR! TRY BEING A COMPULSIVE MASTURBATOR IN A CUBICLE!

VOYEURISM

(AROUSAL FROM WATCHING OTHER PEOPLE DOING SEXY THINGS) AND

EXHIBITIONISM

(AROUSAL FROM SHOWING OFF) ARE BOTH COMMON IN MILD FORM. WE POSE FOR PICTURES, HAVE SEX IN FRONT OF A MIRROR, AND SPEND BILLIONS ON EROTIC VIDEOS, MOVIES, BOOKS, MAGAZINES, WEB SITES...

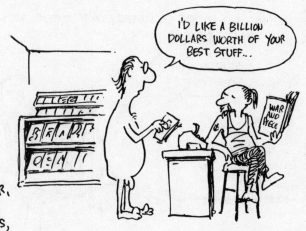

I'D LIKE A BILLION DOLLARS WORTH OF YOUR BEST STUFF...

NO SIGN OF MENTAL IMBALANCE THERE — UNTIL THE VOYEUR BEGINS TO SPY ON UNSUSPECTING VICTIMS, OR THE EXHIBITIONIST BECOMES A FLASHER. THEN IT'S PARAPHILIA, AND ILLEGAL.

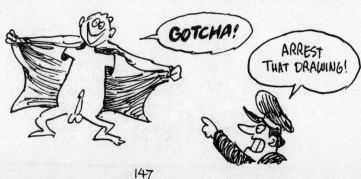

GOTCHA!

ARREST THAT DRAWING!

NONCOERCIVE PARAPHILIAS, ON THE OTHER HAND, ARE USUALLY CONSIDERED HARMLESS, SINCE THEY ARE VICTIMLESS.

FOR EXAMPLE, **FETISHISM** IS THE RITUAL USE OF THINGS — "FETISHES"— AS SEXUAL OBJECTS. MOST FETISHISTS ARE MEN, AND THE FETISHES ARE USUALLY ITEMS OF WOMEN'S CLOTHING SUCH AS SHOES, UNDERWEAR, AND GLOVES.

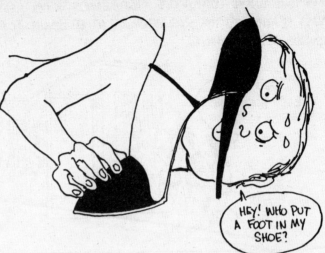

HEY! WHO PUT A FOOT IN MY SHOE?

FETISHISM THAT FOCUSES EXCLUSIVELY ON INDIVIDUAL BODY PARTS — FEET, EARS, BREASTS — IS CALLED **PARTIALISM.**

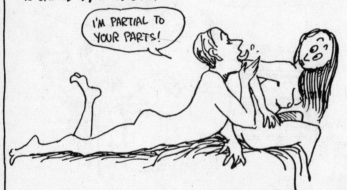

I'M PARTIAL TO YOUR PARTS!

THESE FETISHISTIC RESPONSES MAY BE ROOTED IN CHILDHOOD AND INVOLVE THE TRANSFER OF POWERFUL EROTIC URGES FROM AN IMPORTANT FEMALE TO AN ITEM ASSOCIATED WITH HER.

A MORE DANGEROUS SOLO PURSUIT IS **SELF-STRANGULATION.** SOME PEOPLE DISCOVER THAT ASPHYXIATION ENHANCES ORGASM... AND EVERY YEAR, A FEW OF THEM — MOSTLY BOYS AND YOUNG MEN — GO TOO FAR AND DIE IN THE ACT. **DON'T DO IT!**

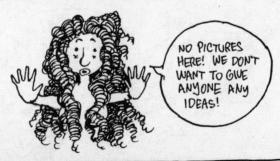

NO PICTURES HERE! WE DON'T WANT TO GIVE ANYONE ANY IDEAS!

OTHER PARAPHILIAS THAT COERCE UNWILLING (OR UNWITTING) VICTIMS ARE **NECROPHILIA** (SEX WITH DEAD PEOPLE) AND **PEDOPHILIA** (SEX WITH CHILDREN).

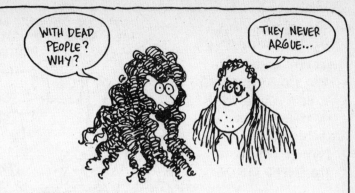

SOME PEDOPHILES, INCIDENTALLY, ROUNDLY INSIST THAT CHILDREN ARE SEXUAL BEINGS WHO SHOULD BE FREE TO HAVE SEX LIKE ANYONE ELSE.

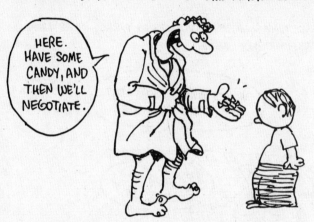

TO THIS, SOCIETY MIGHT WELL RESPOND THAT CHILDREN KNOW HOW TO WRITE, TOO, BUT WE DON'T LET THEM SIGN CONTRACTS!

WHAT MAKES PEOPLE WANT TO PERFORM THESE ACTS? THE ANSWER TO THIS QUESTION IS AS OBSCURE AS THE REASON FOR ANY OTHER MENTAL DISTURBANCE... BUT USUALLY, SOCIETY IGNORES THIS ISSUE AND REGARDS THE BEHAVIOR AS CRIMINAL RATHER THAN A MEDICAL PROBLEM.

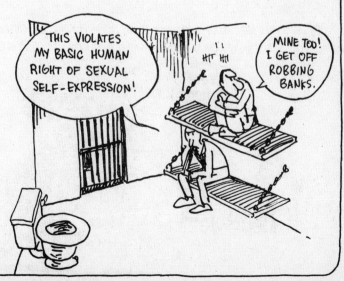

ZOOPHILIA, SEX WITH ANIMALS, IS ALSO USUALLY CONSIDERED TO BE A NONCOERCIVE PARAPHILIA, BUT WE DON'T THINK THE PSYCHOLOGISTS ASKED THE SHEEP'S OPINION.

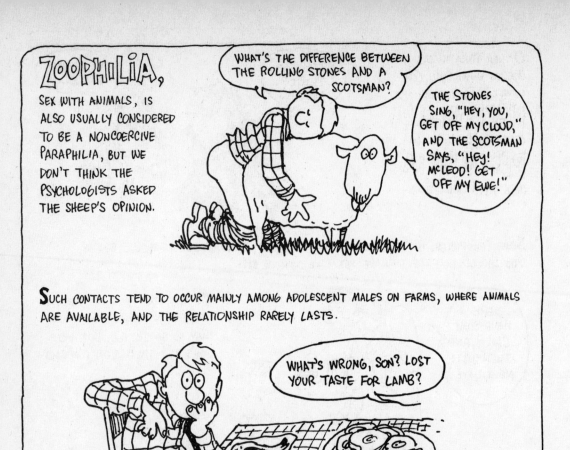

SUCH CONTACTS TEND TO OCCUR MAINLY AMONG ADOLESCENT MALES ON FARMS, WHERE ANIMALS ARE AVAILABLE, AND THE RELATIONSHIP RARELY LASTS.

WELL, THIS WRAPS UP OUR LITTLE TOUR OF SEXUAL EXPRESSION... WE HAVE TO MOVE ON TO OTHER SUBJECTS, EVEN THOUGH THERE'S NO END TO THIS ONE...

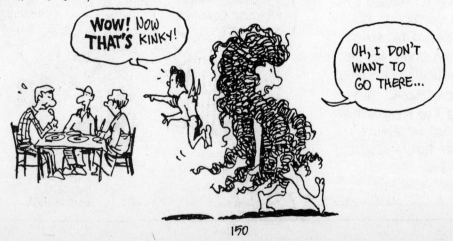

150

··CHAPTER 9··

NOT GETTING PREGNANT

SEXUAL INTERCOURSE IS NATURE'S WAY OF MAKING BABIES... BUT WHAT IF YOU DON'T WANT TO HAVE A BABY AT THIS PARTICULAR TIME?

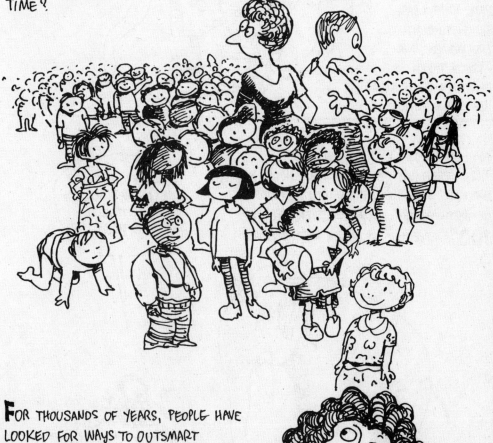

FOR THOUSANDS OF YEARS, PEOPLE HAVE LOOKED FOR WAYS TO OUTSMART MOTHER NATURE.

ANCIENT EGYPTIAN WOMEN FLUSHED THEIR VAGINAS WITH A SUPPOSITORY MADE OF CROCODILE DUNG AND SOUR MILK (THE ACID MIXTURE KILLED SPERM). ELEPHANT DUNG, EVEN MORE ACID, WAS ALSO USED... VAGINAL SPONGES, TO SOAK UP SPERM, DATE TO AT LEAST THE FIFTH CENTURY... AND WOMEN HAVE ALWAYS TAKEN FERTILITY-CONTROLLING HERBS AND POTIONS.

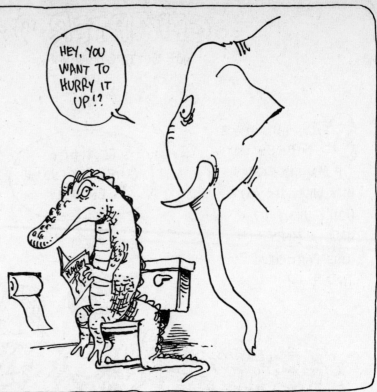

HEY, YOU WANT TO HURRY IT UP!?

NO ONE KNOWS EXACTLY HOW EFFECTIVE THESE PREPARATIONS WERE... BUT NOWADAYS WE HAVE SOME NEW, HIGH-TECH METHODS OF BIRTH CONTROL, SOME OF THEM NEARLY **100%** EFFECTIVE AT PREVENTING PREGNANCY.

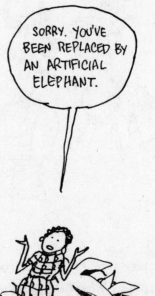

SORRY. YOU'VE BEEN REPLACED BY AN ARTIFICIAL ELEPHANT.

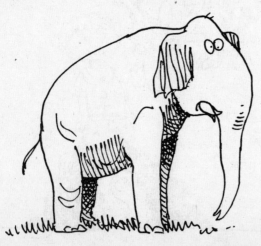

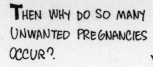

THEN WHY DO SO MANY UNWANTED PREGNANCIES OCCUR?

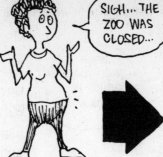

SIGH... THE ZOO WAS CLOSED...

BECAUSE PEOPLE OFTEN USE BIRTH CONTROL INCORRECTLY, INCONSISTENTLY, OR NOT AT ALL.

SEX IS LIKE GAMBLING. EVERY TIME WE PLAY AND WIN, WE FEEL OVERCONFIDENT ABOUT WINNING AGAIN. EVERY TIME WE EMERGE UNPREGNANT FROM UNPROTECTED SEX, IT INCREASES OUR WILLINGNESS TO RUN THE RISK AGAIN... AND THE RISK OF PREGNANCY FROM A SINGLE ENCOUNTER IS ONLY AROUND 3%*

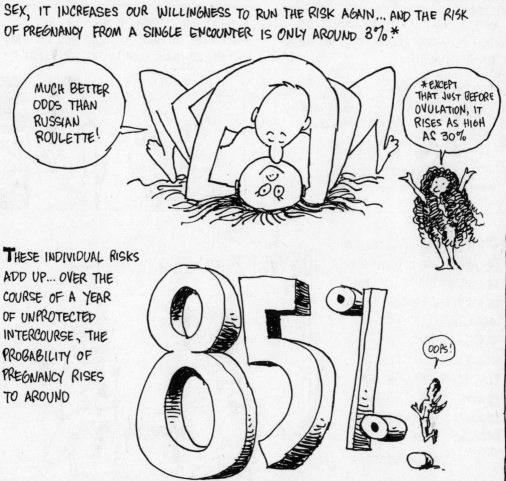

MUCH BETTER ODDS THAN RUSSIAN ROULETTE!

*EXCEPT THAT JUST BEFORE OVULATION, IT RISES AS HIGH AS 30%

THESE INDIVIDUAL RISKS ADD UP... OVER THE COURSE OF A YEAR OF UNPROTECTED INTERCOURSE, THE PROBABILITY OF PREGNANCY RISES TO AROUND 85%

OOPS!

ANOTHER REASON THAT PEOPLE—ESPECIALLY YOUNG PEOPLE—AVOID BIRTH CONTROL IS THAT IT REQUIRES PLANNING.

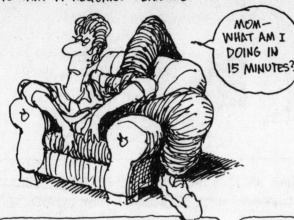

MOM—WHAT AM I DOING IN 15 MINUTES?

THIS IS A SKILL THAT NOT ALL OF US ARE EQUALLY ADEPT AT UNDER THE BEST OF CIRCUMSTANCES, AND WHEN SEX IS INVOLVED, IT'S EVEN HARDER.

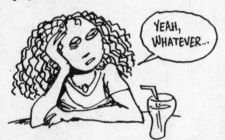

IN THE FIRST PLACE, IT MEANS WE HAVE TO ACKNOWLEDGE OUR INTENTION TO BE SEXUAL.

YEAH, WHATEVER...

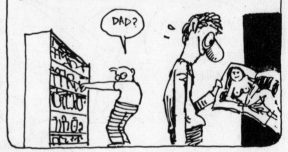

THEN IT MIGHT MEAN A TRIP TO THE MINI-MART TO SHOP FOR CONDOMS, ETC... AND WHO KNOWS WHO MIGHT TURN UP THERE?

DAD?

OR IT INVOLVES CALLING FOR AN APPOINTMENT WITH A DOCTOR OR CLINIC... SITTING IN A PUBLIC WAITING ROOM... ANSWERING PERSONAL QUESTIONS ASKED BY A STRANGER WHO THEN GOES ON TO EXAMINE OUR PRIVATE PARTS... REALLY, IT'S AMAZING THAT ANYBODY USES BIRTH CONTROL!

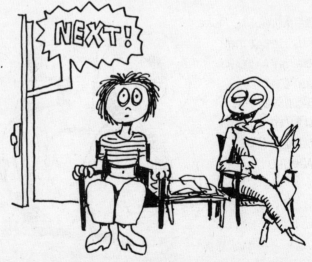

NEXT!

AND BIRTH CONTROL IS UNSPONTANEOUS, A COLD-BLOODED INTERRUPTION OF THE HEAT OF PASSION.

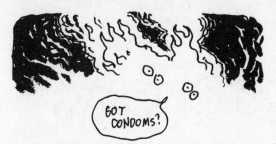

GOT CONDOMS?

ARTIFICIAL BIRTH CONTROL IS AGAINST SOME RELIGIONS.

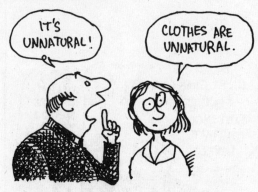

IT'S UNNATURAL!

CLOTHES ARE UNNATURAL.

AND SOME PEOPLE "FORGET" TO USE BIRTH CONTROL BECAUSE THEY SECRETLY OR UNCONSCIOUSLY WANT A BABY.

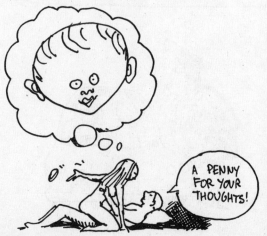

A PENNY FOR YOUR THOUGHTS!

THEN THERE ARE THE REASONS IN FAVOR OF USING BIRTH CONTROL: PREGNANCY AND CHILDBIRTH CARRY SOME RISK... BABIES DEMAND ATTENTION, WORK, TIME, AND MONEY... CHILDREN ARE A LIFELONG COMMITMENT... A BABY THAT'S WANTED WILL BE HAPPIER THAN ONE THAT IS NOT.

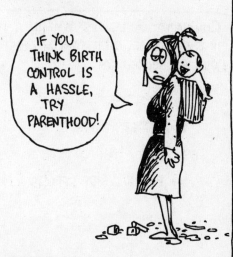

IF YOU THINK BIRTH CONTROL IS A HASSLE, TRY PARENTHOOD!

FOR BOTH THE CHILD AND THE PARENTS, ISN'T IT BETTER TO HAVE BABIES WHEN WE WANT THEM?

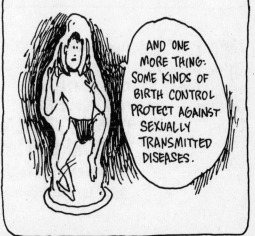

AND ONE MORE THING: SOME KINDS OF BIRTH CONTROL PROTECT AGAINST SEXUALLY TRANSMITTED DISEASES.

SO LET'S ASSUME THE MINOR HASSLE IS WORTH IT... SO NOW IT'S TIME TO LOOK AT SOME OF THE AVAILABLE OPTIONS. THE IDEA BEHIND ALL OF THEM IS THE SAME: TO KEEP SPERM AND EGG FROM GETTING TOGETHER... IN OTHER WORDS, TO PREVENT CONCEPTION... AND SO BIRTH CONTROL IS ALSO CALLED

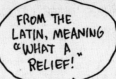

FROM THE LATIN, MEANING "WHAT A RELIEF!"

CONTRACEPTION

CONTRACEPTIVE DEVICES COME IN A DAZZLING VARIETY OF TYPES THAT DIFFER IN CONVENIENCE, COST, COMFORT, AND EFFECTIVENESS. EACH ONE WE DISCUSS WILL BE SCORED ON

* EFFECTIVENESS

* HASSLE FACTOR

* COST

* POSSIBLE SIDE EFFECTS

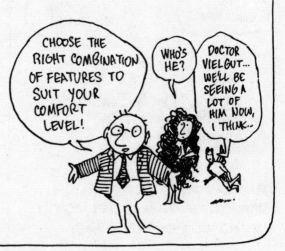

CHOOSE THE RIGHT COMBINATION OF FEATURES TO SUIT YOUR COMFORT LEVEL!

WHO'S HE?

DOCTOR VIELGUT... WE'LL BE SEEING A LOT OF HIM NOW, I THINK...

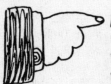

AND REMEMBER: NO CONTRACEPTIVE IS EFFECTIVE IF IT IS NOT USED **CONSISTENTLY** AND **CORRECTLY.** A DIAPHRAGM ACROSS TOWN IS USELESS!!

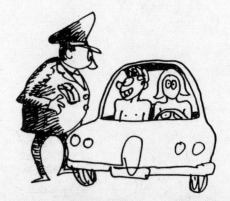

Here are some simple, low-cost, but not necessarily effective methods that people have used over the years.

ABSTINENCE

Not having intercourse is free and 100% effective. It can be a rather challenging option for some people, though.

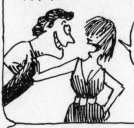

> Like other methods, it must be used consistently to work!

COITUS INTERRUPTUS

"Pulling out" the penis from the vagina before ejaculation can work—sometimes. But mistakes happen, and semen can leak out bf the penis before ejaculation. Unreliable.

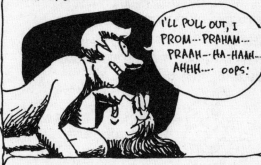

> I'll pull out, I prom—praham— praah—ha-haah— ahhh.... oops!

DOUCHING

Flushing the vagina with liquid is unreliable and unsafe. Sperm may outswim the liquid, and repeated douching messes up vaginal chemistry, leading to irritation and infection.

But if you must, use something slightly acid.

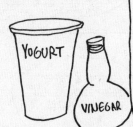

YOGURT

VINEGAR

LACTATION: Breast-feeding suppresses ovulation, but it varies from woman to woman. Unreliable.

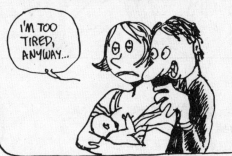

> I'm too tired, anyway...

TOTALLY USELESS

Things to do include: standing up during or after intercourse; jumping up and down, douching with cola, taking one birth-control pill, or using plastic wrap as a condom. Don't even bother!

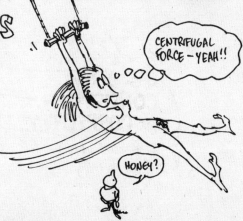

> Centrifugal force—yeah!!

> Honey?

BARRIER METHODS

ALL WORK ON THE SAME PRINCIPLE: PUT SOMETHING BETWEEN SPERM AND EGG.

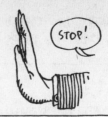

STOP!

HISTORY'S MOST FAMOUS BARRIER METHOD WAS THE **CHASTITY BELT**: A SORT OF METAL UNDERWEAR THAT KNIGHTS USED TO LOCK ONTO THEIR WIVES TO KEEP OTHER KNIGHTS OUT. PRESUMABLY EFFECTIVE, BUT IT CAN'T HAVE DONE MUCH FOR THE MARRIAGE...

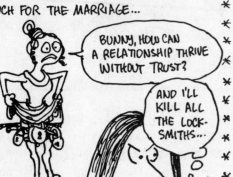

BUNNY, HOW CAN A RELATIONSHIP THRIVE WITHOUT TRUST?

AND I'LL KILL ALL THE LOCK-SMITHS...

PURITAN NEW ENGLAND USED THE **BUNDLING BOARD**, A PLANK THAT WENT DOWN THE CENTER OF THE BED LIKE AN UPSIDE-DOWN KEEL. THE BUNDLING BOARD WAS DESIGNED TO LET UNMARRIED SWEETHEARTS SLEEP TOGETHER WITHOUT "COMPLICATIONS."

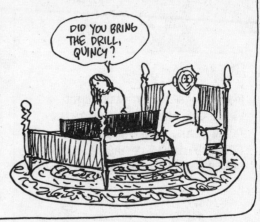

DID YOU BRING THE DRILL, QUINCY?

TODAY'S BARRIERS ARE MADE OF SOFTER, MORE PLIANT STUFF; USUALLY LATEX RUBBER.

LIKE A RUBBER SHEET DOWN THE MIDDLE OF THE BED?

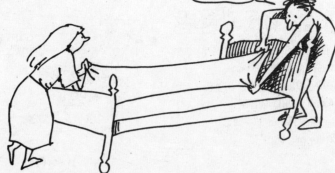

158

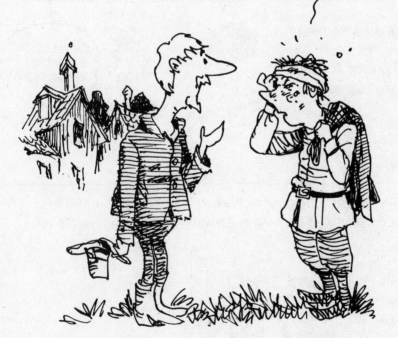

CONDOMS

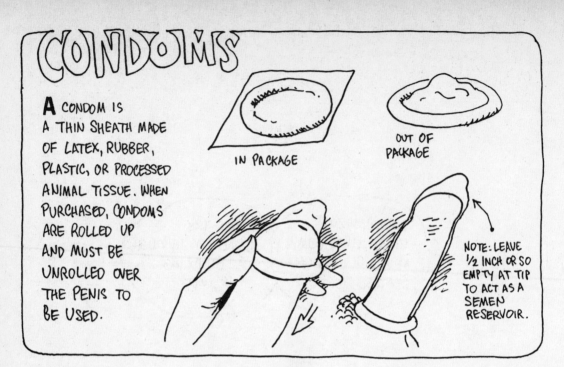

A CONDOM IS A THIN SHEATH MADE OF LATEX, RUBBER, PLASTIC, OR PROCESSED ANIMAL TISSUE. WHEN PURCHASED, CONDOMS ARE ROLLED UP AND MUST BE UNROLLED OVER THE PENIS TO BE USED.

IN PACKAGE

OUT OF PACKAGE

NOTE: LEAVE ½ INCH OR SO EMPTY AT TIP TO ACT AS A SEMEN RESERVOIR.

CONDOMS COME IN AN ASSORTMENT OF SIZES, SHAPES, TEXTURES, AND EVEN FLAVORS... SAMPLE SEVERAL AND SEE WHAT YOU LIKE BEST!

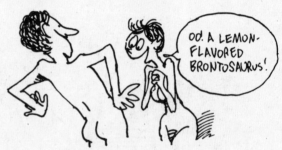

OO. A LEMON-FLAVORED BRONTOSAURUS!

USED CORRECTLY AND CONSISTENTLY, CONDOMS PROVIDE GOOD PROTECTION AGAINST PREGNANCY. LATEX CONDOMS ALSO HELP DETER SEXUALLY TRANSMITTED DISEASES (STDs).

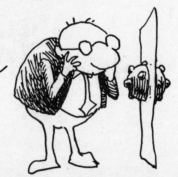

NOTE: USE LATEX ONLY!!! VIRUSES CAN PASS THROUGH LAMBSKIN CONDOMS!

EFFECTIVENESS: MODERATE TO HIGH
HASSLE FACTOR: LOW TO MEDIUM
COST: LOW
SIDE EFFECTS: NONE

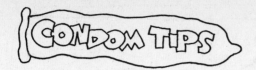
CONDOM TIPS

USE CONDOMS EVERY TIME. CONSISTENCY IS THE KEY TO EFFECTIVENESS!

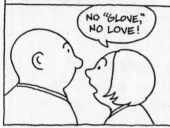

NO "GLOVE," NO LOVE!

USE LATEX OR POLYURETHANE (PLASTIC) CONDOMS. THEY PROTECT AGAINST STDS.

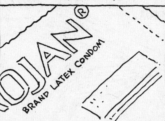

USE CONDOMS THAT CONTAIN A SPERMICIDE, OR USE THEM WITH A SEPARATE SPERMICIDE.

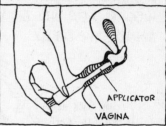

APPLICATOR

VAGINA

PUT ON THE CONDOM BEFORE THE PENIS COMES NEAR ANY BODY OPENING.

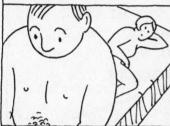

LEAVE ½ INCH OF SPACE AT THE TIP. DO NOT BLOW AIR INTO THE CONDOM.

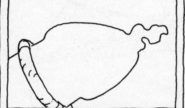

SOON AFTER EJACULATION, HOLD THE BASE OF THE CONDOM SECURELY AGAINST THE PENIS AND WITHDRAW THE PENIS FROM THE VAGINA OR OTHER ORIFICE.

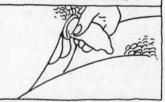

AFTER USE, CHECK THE CONDOM FOR TEARS OR HOLES.

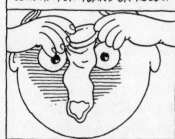

IF YOU FIND A LEAK, IMMEDIATELY INSERT SPERMICIDE INTO THE VAGINA.

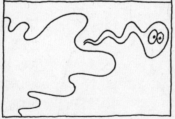

IF BROKEN CONDOMS ARE A PERSISTENT PROBLEM, TRY USING A WATER-BASED LUBRICANT TO REDUCE FRICTION, OR TRY A DIFFERENT BRAND OF CONDOM.

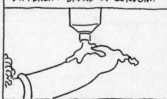

DO NOT REUSE CONDOMS!

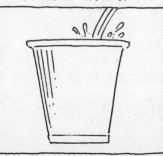

KEEP OIL-BASED PRODUCTS LIKE PETROLEUM JELLY AWAY FROM CONDOMS. THEY CAN CAUSE THE LATEX TO DETERIORATE.

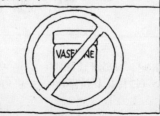

STORE CONDOMS IN A COOL, DRY, CONVENIENT PLACE. IT'S OKAY TO CARRY A CONDOM IN YOUR WALLET, BUT NOT FOR MORE THAN TWO WEEKS.

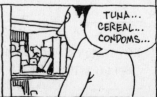

TUNA... CEREAL... CONDOMS...

THE DIAPHRAGM

IS A BARRIER METHOD FOR FEMALES; A RUBBER CUP WITH A FLEXIBLE RIM, INSERTED DEEP INTO THE VAGINA, AGAINST THE CERVIX.

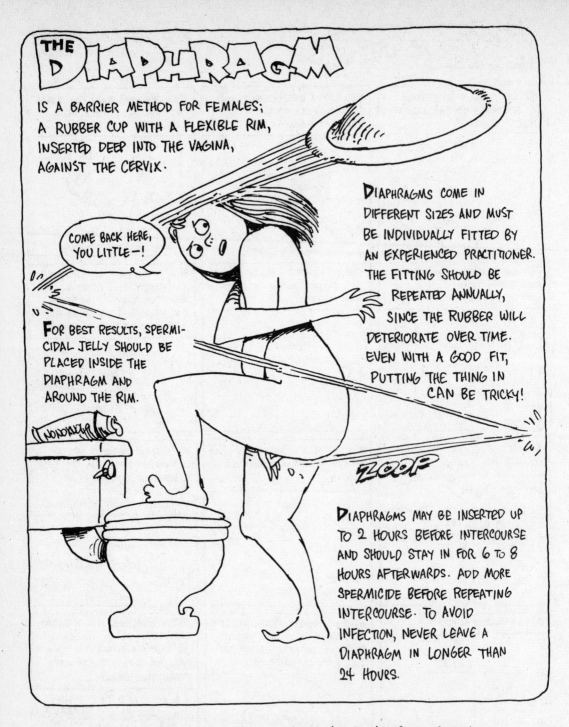

COME BACK HERE, YOU LITTLE—!

FOR BEST RESULTS, SPERMICIDAL JELLY SHOULD BE PLACED INSIDE THE DIAPHRAGM AND AROUND THE RIM.

DIAPHRAGMS COME IN DIFFERENT SIZES AND MUST BE INDIVIDUALLY FITTED BY AN EXPERIENCED PRACTITIONER. THE FITTING SHOULD BE REPEATED ANNUALLY, SINCE THE RUBBER WILL DETERIORATE OVER TIME. EVEN WITH A GOOD FIT, PUTTING THE THING IN CAN BE TRICKY!

ZOOP

DIAPHRAGMS MAY BE INSERTED UP TO 2 HOURS BEFORE INTERCOURSE AND SHOULD STAY IN FOR 6 TO 8 HOURS AFTERWARDS. ADD MORE SPERMICIDE BEFORE REPEATING INTERCOURSE. TO AVOID INFECTION, NEVER LEAVE A DIAPHRAGM IN LONGER THAN 24 HOURS.

EFFECTIVENESS: MODERATE TO HIGH; HASSLE FACTOR: LOW TO MODERATE; COST: LOW; SIDE EFFECTS: RARE; A BADLY FITTED DIAPHRAGM CAN CAUSE DISCOMFORT.

MORE BARRIERS

THE **CERVICAL CAP** IS A SMALL RUBBER GIZMO THAT FITS SNUGLY OVER THE CERVIX. IT MUST BE INDIVIDUALLY FITTED BY A DOCTOR OR CLINICIAN.

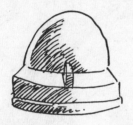

THE **FEMALE CONDOM** IS A SOFT, LOOSE-FITTING POLYURETHANE SHEATH. ONE END IS A BARRIER THAT FITS OVER THE CERVIX. THE OTHER END IS AN OPEN RING THAT STAYS JUST OUTSIDE THE VAGINA.

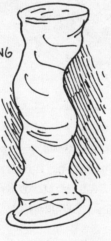

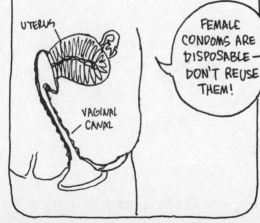

UTERUS

VAGINAL CANAL

FEMALE CONDOMS ARE DISPOSABLE— DON'T REUSE THEM!

BARRIER METHODS ARE MORE EFFECTIVE WHEN COMBINED WITH A

SPERMICIDE,

A SUBSTANCE TOXIC TO SPERM. WHETHER IT TAKES THE FORM OF A JELLY, FOAM, CREAM, TABLET, OR SUPPOSITORY, THE PRINCIPLE IS ALWAYS THE SAME:

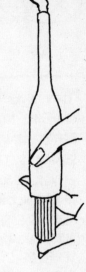

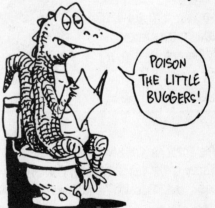

POISON THE LITTLE BUGGERS!

SPERMICIDES CAN ALSO KILL SEVERAL KINDS OF DISEASE-CAUSING ORGANISMS. AND SO REDUCE THE RISK OF SOME STDs. BUT THEY ARE NOT FOOLPROOF AND SHOULD NOT BE RELIED ON AS YOUR ONLY METHOD OF DISEASE PREVENTION.

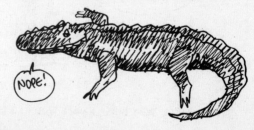

NOPE!

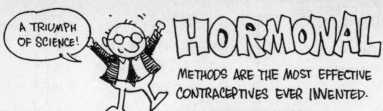

HORMONAL

A TRIUMPH OF SCIENCE!

METHODS ARE THE MOST EFFECTIVE CONTRACEPTIVES EVER INVENTED.

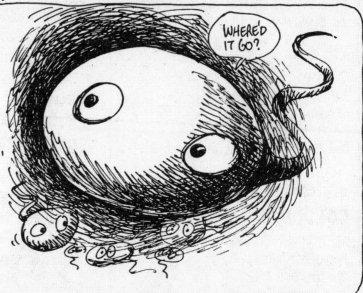

THEY WORK BY CHANGING A WOMAN'S REPRODUCTIVE CYCLE. HORMONES, TAKEN EITHER ORALLY, BY INJECTION, OR FROM TIME-RELEASE IMPLANTS, ALTER A WOMAN'S LEVEL OF ESTROGEN AND PROGESTERONE TO PREVENT OVULATION. SPERM AND EGG CAN'T GET TOGETHER IF THERE IS NO EGG!

WHERE'D IT GO?

ONE POPULAR HORMONAL METHOD IS THE ORAL CONTRACEPTIVE, OR PILLoooo A SERIES OF PILLS, REALLY, CONTAINING ESTROGEN AND/OR PROGESTERONE. A WOMAN TAKES ONE PILL EVERY MORNING FOR 20 OR 21 DAYS, FOLLOWED BY A WEEK OFF. IF SHE FORGETS TO TAKE A PILL, SHE TAKES TWO THE FOLLOWING DAY.

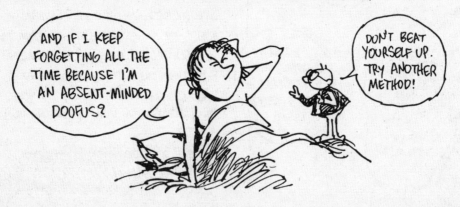

AND IF I KEEP FORGETTING ALL THE TIME BECAUSE I'M AN ABSENT-MINDED DOOFUS?

DON'T BEAT YOURSELF UP. TRY ANOTHER METHOD!

EFFECTIVENESS: VERY HIGH; HASSLE FACTOR: MODERATE; COST: MODERATE; SIDE EFFECTS: SEE BELOW.

164

IMPLANTS,

UNDER THE BRAND NAME NORPLANT, ARE TIME-RELEASED SYNTHETIC PROGESTERONE IN THE FORM OF SMALL STICKS. SIX OF THEM ARE INSERTED UNDER THE SKIN OF A WOMAN'S ARM, WHERE THEY LEAK OUT HORMONES THAT PREVENT PREGNANCY FOR 5 YEARS. FERTILITY CAN BE RESTORED BY REMOVING THE IMPLANTS, BUT THE REMOVAL MUST BE DONE BY A CLINICIAN.

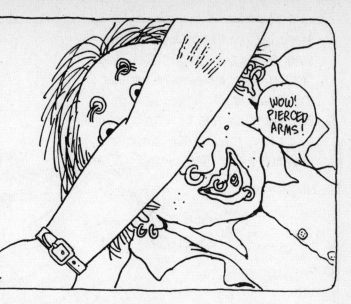

WOW! PIERCED ARMS!

DEPO-PROVERA (OR DMPA) IS GIVEN AS A SINGLE INJECTION THAT PREVENTS PREGNANCY FOR 3 MONTHS. IT ALSO STOPS MENSTRUATION AT THE SAME TIME.

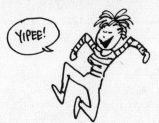

YIPEE!

DMPA IS HEAVY-DUTY STUFF AND CAN REDUCE FERTILITY FOR AS LONG AS A YEAR AFTER THE INJECTIONS STOP.

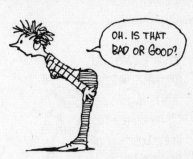

OH. IS THAT BAD OR GOOD?

WARNING:

ALL HORMONAL CONTRACEPTIVES CARRY CERTAIN HEALTH RISKS: THE PILL, FOR INSTANCE, SLIGHTLY INCREASES A WOMAN'S CHANCE OF STROKE, BLOOD CLOTTING, AND HEART ATTACK. WOMEN OVER 35, SMOKERS, AND WOMEN WITH HEART PROBLEMS MAY WANT TO AVOID THE PILL. IT IS IMPORTANT TO REMEMBER, HOWEVER, THAT FOR MOST WOMEN, THE PILL IS SAFER THAN PREGNANCY.

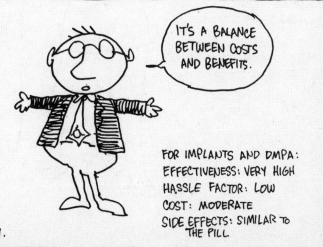

IT'S A BALANCE BETWEEN COSTS AND BENEFITS.

FOR IMPLANTS AND DMPA:
EFFECTIVENESS: VERY HIGH
HASSLE FACTOR: LOW
COST: MODERATE
SIDE EFFECTS: SIMILAR TO THE PILL

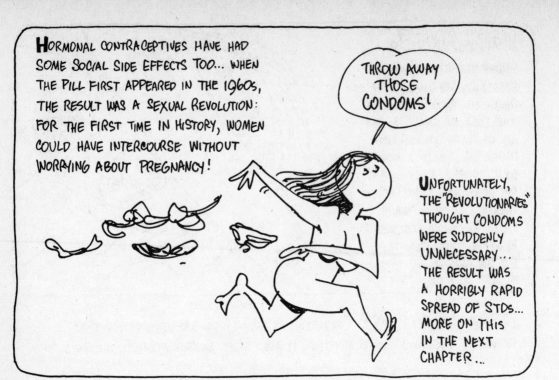

HORMONAL CONTRACEPTIVES HAVE HAD SOME SOCIAL SIDE EFFECTS TOO... WHEN THE PILL FIRST APPEARED IN THE 1960s, THE RESULT WAS A SEXUAL REVOLUTION: FOR THE FIRST TIME IN HISTORY, WOMEN COULD HAVE INTERCOURSE WITHOUT WORRYING ABOUT PREGNANCY!

THROW AWAY THOSE CONDOMS!

UNFORTUNATELY, THE "REVOLUTIONARIES" THOUGHT CONDOMS WERE SUDDENLY UNNECESSARY... THE RESULT WAS A HORRIBLY RAPID SPREAD OF STDs... MORE ON THIS IN THE NEXT CHAPTER...

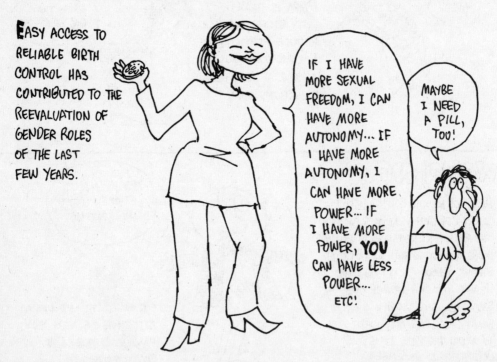

EASY ACCESS TO RELIABLE BIRTH CONTROL HAS CONTRIBUTED TO THE REEVALUATION OF GENDER ROLES OF THE LAST FEW YEARS.

IF I HAVE MORE SEXUAL FREEDOM, I CAN HAVE MORE AUTONOMY... IF I HAVE MORE AUTONOMY, I CAN HAVE MORE POWER... IF I HAVE MORE POWER, **YOU** CAN HAVE LESS POWER... ETC!

MAYBE I NEED A PILL, TOO!

AT THE SAME TIME, HORMONAL CONTRACEPTION SEEMED TO REINFORCE THE IDEA THAT BIRTH CONTROL IS ALL THE FEMALE'S RESPONSIBILTTY.

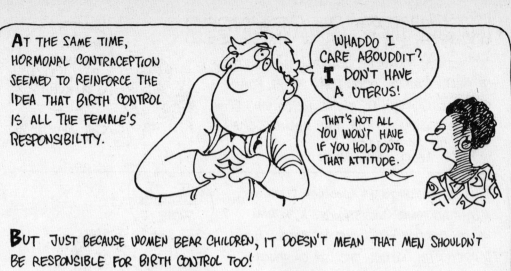

BUT JUST BECAUSE WOMEN BEAR CHILDREN, IT DOESN'T MEAN THAT MEN SHOULDN'T BE RESPONSIBLE FOR BIRTH CONTROL TOO!

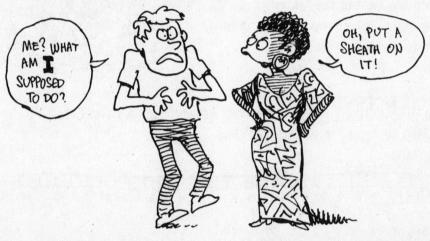

AT THE VERY LEAST, MEN CAN SHARE RESPONSIBILITY BY BUYING AND USING CONDOMS. THEY CAN ALSO HELP PAY THE COSTS OF CLINIC BILLS, PILLS, SPERMICIDES, AND OTHER SUPPLIES.

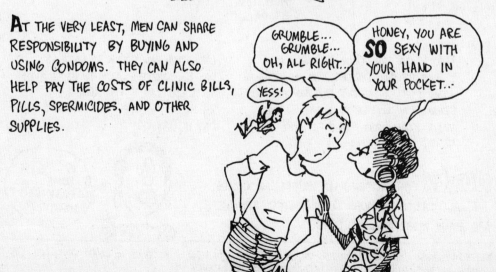

FERTILITY AWARENESS

OR "NATURAL FAMILY PLANNING" IS A METHOD OF BIRTH CONTROL ACCEPTABLE TO THE ROMAN CATHOLIC CHURCH. IT MEANS REFRAINING FROM INTERCOURSE DURING THE TIME WHEN A WOMAN IS KNOWN TO BE FERTILE.

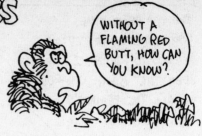

THIS METHOD REQUIRES EDUCATION, PLANNING, MOTIVATION, AND PERSISTENCE. A WOMAN HAS TO MONITOR HER CYCLE ACCURATELY AND CONSISTENTLY, NOTING THE DAY ON WHICH HER PERIOD BEGAN, THE NUMBER OF DAYS UNTIL THE NEXT PERIOD, AND ANY VARIATION IN THE TIME BETWEEN PERIODS.

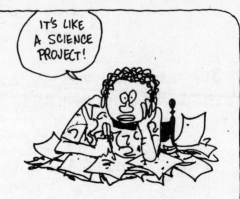

THE **CALENDAR**, OR RHYTHM, METHOD GOES BY THE CALENDAR. FOR A 28-DAY CYCLE, IT WORKS LIKE THIS:

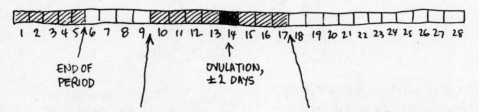

1 2 3 4 5 6 7 8 9 10 11 12 13 14 15 16 17 18 19 20 21 22 23 24 25 26 27 28

END OF PERIOD

OVULATION, ±2 DAYS

OVULATION CAN OCCUR AS EARLY AS 16 DAYS BEFORE THE ONSET OF MENSTRUATION (I.E., ON DAY 12), BUT SINCE SPERM CAN LIVE UP TO 2 DAYS IN THE VAGINA, THE FIRST "UNSAFE" DAY IS DAY 10.

OVULATION CAN OCCUR AS LATE AS DAY 16, AND THE OVUM IS RECEPTIVE TO FERTILIZATION FOR ABOUT 24 HOURS, SO THE FINAL UNSAFE DAY IS DAY 17.

NOTE: FOR WOMEN WITH IRREGULAR CYCLES, THE CALCULATION IS MORE COMPLICATED, AND THERE ARE MANY MORE UNSAFE DAYS.

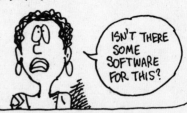

EFFECTIVENESS: VARIABLE, DEPENDING ON THE INDIVIDUAL; GENERALLY MODERATE TO LOW; COST: ZERO; HASSLE FACTOR: MODERATE; SIDE EFFECTS: ONLY PREGNANCY

FOR FURTHER CLUES, A WOMAN CAN MONITOR HER TEMPERATURE EVERY DAY AT THE SAME TIME, USUALLY FIRST THING IN THE MORNING. THIS **BASAL BODY TEMPERATURE** RISES ABOUT ½ TO 1 DEGREE (FAHRENHEIT) AT OVULATION AND STAYS HIGH UNTIL THE NEXT PERIOD.

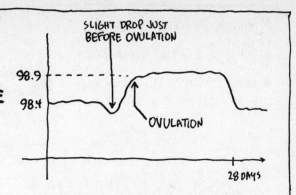

SLIGHT DROP JUST BEFORE OVULATION

98.9
98.4

OVULATION

28 DAYS

ONCE SHE DETERMINES HER PATTERN — IF THERE IS ONE! — A WOMAN CAN ABSTAIN FROM INTERCOURSE STARTING 3 TO 4 DAYS BEFORE THE EXPECTED RISE AND RESUME ONLY 4 DAYS AFTER THE RISE HAS OCCURRED.

ALSO: AT OVULATION, CERVICAL MUCUS, WHICH IS DISCHARGED FROM THE VAGINA, BECOMES CLEAR, SLIPPERY, AND ELASTIC, SIMILAR TO RAW EGG WHITE.

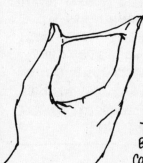

A DROP CAN BE STRETCHED BETWEEN THE FINGERS, LIKE THIS.

THE 4 DAYS BEFORE AND 4 DAYS AFTER THIS ELASTICITY BEGINS ARE CONSIDERED UNSAFE.

ANOTHER SIGN OF OVULATION IS **MITTELSCHMERZ**, A MID-CYCLE ABDOMINAL PAIN.

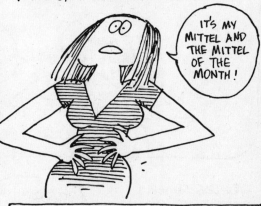

IT'S MY MITTEL AND THE MITTEL OF THE MONTH!

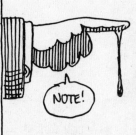

NOTE!

ALL THESE METHODS CALCULATE BACK FROM THE BEGINNING OF THE **NEXT** PERIOD. THIS MAKES THEM ESPECIALLY INEFFECTIVE FOR WOMEN WITH IRREGULAR CYCLES, INCLUDING NURSING MOTHERS.

ON THE OTHER HAND, THEY WORK PRETTY WELL IF YOU'RE TRYING TO GET PREGNANT: JUST USE THE RHYTHM METHOD IN REVERSE!!

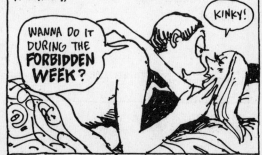

WANNA DO IT DURING THE **FORBIDDEN WEEK**?

KINKY!

IN A CLASS BY ITSELF IS THE **IUD** (**I**ntra**U**terine **D**evice), A SMALL COPPER OR PLASTIC DEVICE THAT IS INSERTED INTO THE UTERUS.

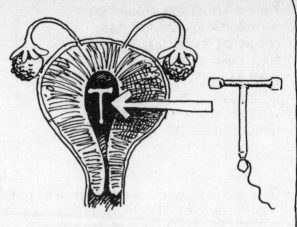

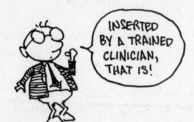

INSERTED BY A TRAINED CLINICIAN, THAT IS!

WARNING: NOT ALL IUDs ARE ALIKE. SOME SHAPES AND MATERIALS CAN BE VERY IRRITATING, CAUSING CRAMPS, EXTRA-HEAVY MENSTRUAL FLOW, PELVIC INFLAMMATORY DISEASE (ESPECIALLY IN WOMEN WITH MULTIPLE PARTNERS), SCARRING OF THE UTERUS, AND INFERTILITY.

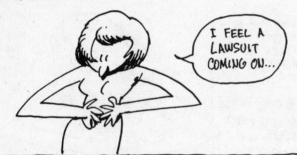

I FEEL A LAWSUIT COMING ON...

THESE PROBLEMS PROMPTED SO MANY WOMEN TO SUE THE IUD MANUFACTURERS THAT THE DEVICE WAS MOSTLY PULLED OFF THE MARKET. ONE, THE COPPER T-380A, IS STILL AVAILABLE IN THE U.S.

IN LESS LAWYERLY SOCIETIES, THE IUD IS STILL THE CHOICE OF ABOUT **70 MILLION** WOMEN.

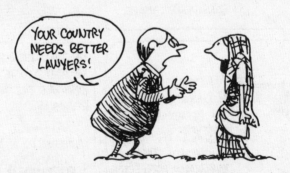

YOUR COUNTRY NEEDS BETTER LAWYERS!

THE STRANGEST THING ABOUT IUDs IS THAT NOBODY KNOWS EXACTLY HOW THEY WORK!

EFFECTIVENESS: HIGH; HASSLE FACTOR: LOW; COST: LOW; SIDE-EFFECTS: SOMETIMES

FINALLY, FOR THOSE WHO WANT PERMANENT BIRTH CONTROL, THERE'S ALWAYS

STERILIZATION.

ABOUT A MILLION AMERICANS GO UNDER THE KNIFE EVERY YEAR.

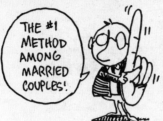

THE #1 METHOD AMONG MARRIED COUPLES!

FOR WOMEN, THE MOST COMMON PROCEDURE IS

TUBAL LIGATION,

WHICH INVOLVES CUTTING OR CAUTERIZING THE FALLOPIAN TUBES.

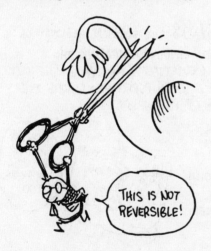

THIS IS NOT REVERSIBLE!

TUBAL LIGATION REQUIRES A SHORT HOSPITAL STAY AND SEVERAL DAYS OF RECOVERY AT HOME.

IN MALE STERILIZATION, OR

VASECTOMY, THE

DOCTOR SNIPS AND TIES OFF THE TWO SPERM DUCTS KNOWN AS THE VASA DEFERENTIA. THIS SIMPLE OPERATION CAN BE DONE IN AN OFFICE VISIT, AND RECOVERY IS QUICK.

NOTE: VASECTOMIES DO NOT AFFECT AROUSAL, ERECTION, OR SEXUAL FUNCTION!

YOU MEAN, I CAN STILL PERFORM LIKE A SCALLION?

DESPITE THE EXTRA TROUBLE AND EXPENSE, WOMEN ELECT TO HAVE TUBAL LIGATIONS ABOUT TWICE AS OFTEN AS MEN OPT FOR VASECTOMY. WE SUSPECT THIS IS BECAUSE WOMEN ARE MORE SURE ABOUT WHEN THEY'VE HAD ENOUGH.

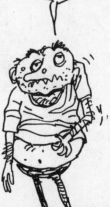

YES, A TROPHY WIFE MAY YET BE MINE!

FINALLY, WE COME TO THE MOST CONTROVERSIAL KIND OF BIRTH CONTROL: THE KIND THAT'S USED AFTER CONCEPTION MAY HAVE ALREADY HAPPENED.

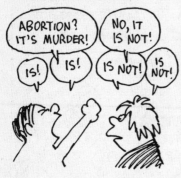

ABORTION? IT'S MURDER!

NO, IT IS NOT!

IS!

IS!

IS NOT!

IS NOT!

WE ARE GOING TO STAY OUT OF THIS ARGUMENT, EXCEPT TO SAY ONE THING: AT THIS WRITING, ABORTIONS ARE LEGAL, AND SHOOTING DOCTORS WHO PERFORM THEM IS NOT.

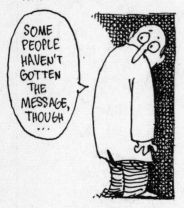

SOME PEOPLE HAVEN'T GOTTEN THE MESSAGE, THOUGH...

WITHOUT FURTHER ADO, HERE ARE THREE POST-COITAL OPTIONS.

ECPs ("EMERGENCY CONTRACEPTIVE PILLS"): ORDINARY BIRTH CONTROL PILLS CAN BE TAKEN IN HIGH DOSAGE WITHIN 72 HOURS AFTER UNPROTECTED INTERCOURSE. THIS INDUCES THE UTERUS TO SHED ITS LINING.

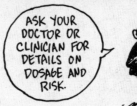

ASK YOUR DOCTOR OR CLINICIAN FOR DETAILS ON DOSAGE AND RISK.

RU 486 (OR MIFEPRISTONE):

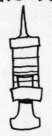

A STEROID TAKEN BY INJECTION, RU486 MAY BE USED TO INDUCE MISCARRIAGE WITHIN THE FIRST 5-6 WEEKS OF PREGNANCY. MAINLY USED IN EUROPE, IT IS STILL NOT WIDELY AVAILABLE IN THE U.S.

ABORTION: THE SURGICAL REMOVAL OF AN EMBRYO USUALLY INVOLVES SCRAPING THE UTERINE LINING ("CURETTAGE") AND VACUUMING OUT THE TISSUE. SAFEST WHEN PERFORMED DURING THE FIRST 3 MONTHS OF PREGNANCY.

ABORTION CARRIES A CERTAIN HEALTH RISK, WHICH IS MINIMIZED BY DOING IT IN A SANITARY MEDICAL ENVIRONMENT WITH QUALIFIED PEOPLE.

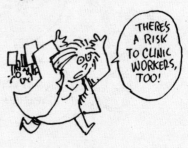

THERE'S A RISK TO CLINIC WORKERS, TOO!

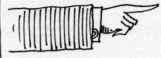

21% OF AMERICAN WOMEN OF REPRODUCTIVE AGE HAVE HAD AT LEAST ONE ABORTION.

As you can see, no contraceptive is ideal: the most effective ones may have side effects, while the medically safest ones are neither hassle-free nor error-proof. What is science doing to improve the situation?

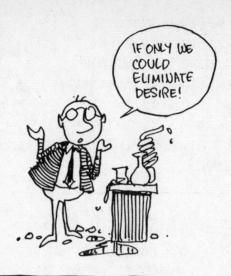

Some current areas of active research:

Refining existing hormonal methods to reduce or eliminate side-effects.

Inventing new surgical gimmicks like tiny plugs and clips that would make sterilization reversible.

Developing a male birth-control pill that doesn't make you sick. (So far, they all do.)

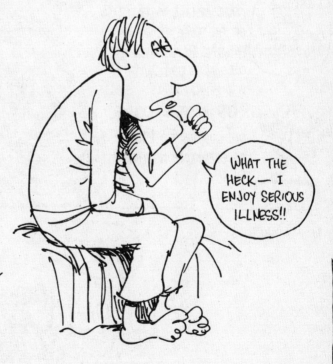

SINCE NO CURRENT METHOD IS PERFECT, CHOOSING THE "RIGHT" CONTRACEPTIVE IS A PERSONAL DECISION, BALANCING THE FACTORS OF COMFORT, CONVENIENCE, COST, AND EFFECTIVENESS. (AND DON'T FORGET THE COST AND INCONVENIENCE OF PREGNANCY!)

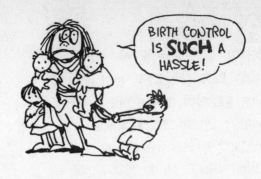

BIRTH CONTROL IS **SUCH** A HASSLE!

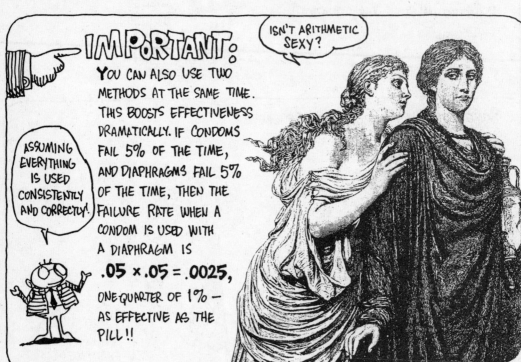

IMPORTANT:

YOU CAN ALSO USE TWO METHODS AT THE SAME TIME. THIS BOOSTS EFFECTIVENESS DRAMATICALLY. IF CONDOMS FAIL 5% OF THE TIME, AND DIAPHRAGMS FAIL 5% OF THE TIME, THEN THE FAILURE RATE WHEN A CONDOM IS USED WITH A DIAPHRAGM IS

$$.05 \times .05 = .0025,$$

ONE QUARTER OF 1% — AS EFFECTIVE AS THE PILL!!

ASSUMING EVERYTHING IS USED CONSISTENTLY AND CORRECTLY!

ISN'T ARITHMETIC SEXY?

OUR ADVICE IS —

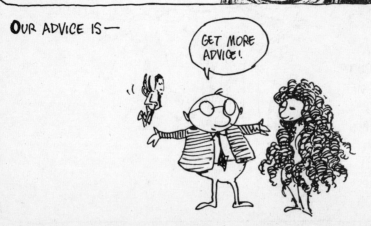

GET MORE ADVICE!

174

···°°CHAPTER 10°°°°

SEXUAL HEALTH
AND THE ALTERNATIVE...

THESE DAYS, MESSAGES ABOUT SEXUAL HEALTH ARE HARD TO IGNORE... THEY'RE EVERYWHERE... BUT FOR SOME REASON, A LOT OF US AREN'T GETTING THE MESSAGE UNTIL IT'S TOO LATE...

IN THIS CHAPTER, OUR ATTENDING PHYSICIAN **DR. VIELGUT,** HELPS US DISCUSS THE MEDICAL SIDE OF SEXUALITY...

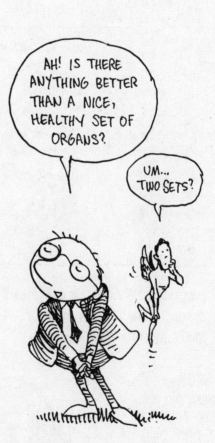

AH! IS THERE ANYTHING BETTER THAN A NICE, HEALTHY SET OF ORGANS?

UM... TWO SETS?

THE FIRST LINE OF DEFENSE IN PROTECTING SEXUAL HEALTH IS TO HAVE GOOD HEALTH HABITS IN GENERAL: EATING WELL, GETTING ENOUGH REST AND EXERCISE, AND KEEPING TOXIC SUBSTANCES OUT OF OUR BODIES.

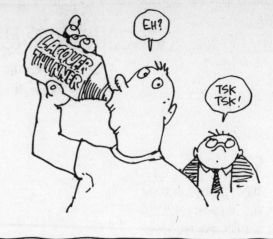

PREVENTION ALSO INCLUDES:

GETTING REGULAR MEDICAL EXAMS...

EVEN IF YOU DON'T LIKE BEING PRRROBED!

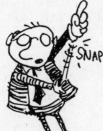

SNAP!

DOING SELF-EXAMS...

DON'T BE SQUEAMISH! USE A MIRROR!

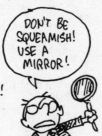

AND BEING AWARE OF SEXUAL-HEALTH ISSUES.

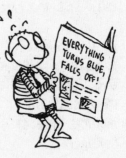

EVERYTHING TURNS BLUE, FALLS OFF!

IT ALSO INVOLVES KNOWING SAFER SEX PRACTICES, KNOWING HOW TO GUARD AGAINST INFECTION BY SEXUALLY TRANSMITTED DISEASES — **STD**s — AND KNOWING SOMETHING ABOUT THEIR SYMPTOMS AND TREATMENT.

IN OTHER WORDS, YOU NEED TO BE A LITTLE BIT YOUR OWN DOCTOR!

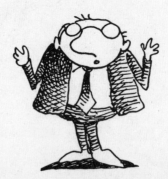

NOT ALL SEXUAL DISEASES ARE SEXUALLY TRANSMITTED. **CANCER,** FOR EXAMPLE, CAN APPEAR IN SEX ORGANS WITHOUT BEING THE RESULT OF SEXUAL CONTACT.* EARLY DETECTION IS THE KEY TO STOPPING MANY KINDS OF CANCER.

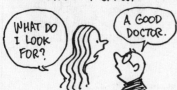

WHAT DO I LOOK FOR?

A GOOD DOCTOR.

CANCER IS MAINLY A DISEASE OF OLDER PEOPLE, BUT EVEN YOUNG WOMEN SHOULD HAVE YEARLY GYNECOLOGICAL EXAMS, INCLUDING A PAP SMEAR TO LOOK FOR CERVICAL CANCER. IN THIS TEST, A FEW CELLS ARE REMOVED FROM THE CERVIX AND EXAMINED UNDER A MICROSCOPE.

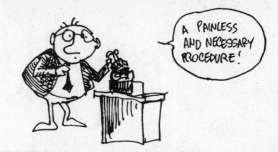

A PAINLESS AND NECESSARY PROCEDURE!

WOMEN SHOULD ALSO GET REGULAR BREAST EXAMS: EVERY 3 YEARS FOR WOMEN UNDER 40, EVERY 2 YEARS, INCLUDING A MAMMOGRAM BETWEEN 40 AND 50, AND ANNUALLY OVER 50.

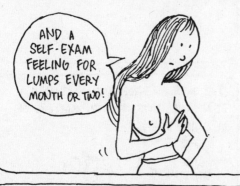

AND A SELF-EXAM FEELING FOR LUMPS EVERY MONTH OR TWO!

GUYS NEED TO CHECK THEMSELVES OUT, TOO. TESTICULAR CANCER IS ON THE RISE, ESPECIALLY AMONG YOUNG WHITE MEN. A SIMPLE SELF-CHECK CAN REVEAL ANY UNUSUAL SWELLING OR LUMPS.

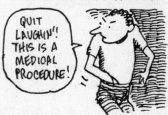

QUIT LAUGHIN'! THIS IS A MEDICAL PROCEDURE!

MEN OVER 40 NEED TO HAVE REGULAR EXAMS FOR PROSTATE CANCER. BECAUSE THIS INVOLVES AN UNCOMFORTABLE RECTAL PROBE, MANY MEN DON'T WANT TO DO IT.

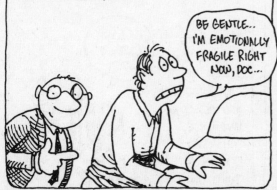

BE GENTLE... I'M EMOTIONALLY FRAGILE RIGHT NOW, DOC...

AVOIDING THIS EXAM IS **STUPID!** PROSTATE CANCER IS SECOND ONLY TO LUNG CANCER AS A KILLER OF MALES, BUT IT HAS A HIGH CURE RATE IF DETECTED EARLY. THE SAME IS TRUE OF TESTICULAR CANCER.

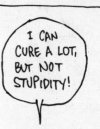

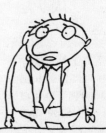

I CAN CURE A LOT, BUT NOT STUPIDITY!

*BUT SOME STDs DO INCREASE THE RISK OF CANCER. SEE BELOW.

FOR YOUNGER PEOPLE, THE MAIN HEALTH CONCERN IS INFECTIOUS DISEASE, WHICH PASSES FROM PERSON TO PERSON, BORNE BY MICROORGANISMS LIKE BACTERIA, VIRUSES, AND YEAST.

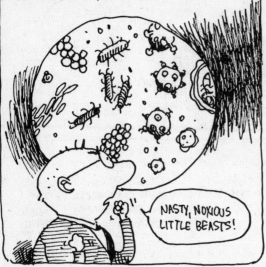

NASTY, NOXIOUS LITTLE BEASTS!

EVERYONE WHO HAS MORE THAN ONE PARTNER — OR WHOSE PARTNER HAS MORE THAN ONE PARTNER — SHOULD BE REGULARLY TESTED FOR STDs, HIV IN PARTICULAR.

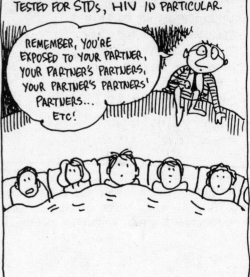

REMEMBER, YOU'RE EXPOSED TO YOUR PARTNER, YOUR PARTNER'S PARTNERS, YOUR PARTNER'S PARTNERS' PARTNERS... ETC!

THINK THERE'S NOT MUCH RISK? THE UNITED STATES IS IN THE THROES OF AN STD EPIDEMIC, WITH OVER **12 MILLION** NEW CASES A YEAR — 2/3 OF THEM IN PEOPLE UNDER 25.

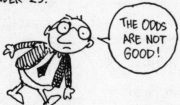

THE ODDS ARE NOT GOOD!

WHEN YOU ADD IT UP, AT LEAST **10%** OF YOUNG PEOPLE AGED 16-24 WILL BE INFECTED ANNUALLY — AND PERHAPS HALF CAN EXPECT TO HAVE AN STD SOMETIME DURING THEIR LIVES.

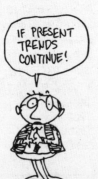

IF PRESENT TRENDS CONTINUE!

THE HASSLES INVOLVED RANGE FROM LOW-LEVEL NUISANCES TO MATTERS OF LIFE AND DEATH.

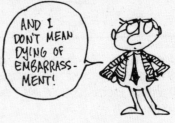

AND I DON'T MEAN DYING OF EMBARRASS-MENT!

NOW WE'RE GOING TO TAKE A TOUR OF THESE PARASITES, AND WE SHOULD WARN YOU, THIS ISN'T EXACTLY A TURN-ON...

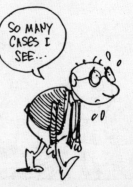

SO MANY CASES I SEE...

CHLAMYDIA

THE MOST COMMON OF ALL, AND OFTEN GOES UNTREATED BECAUSE IT HAS NO SYMPTOMS.

O CHLAMYDIA TRACHOMATIS, A VIRUSLIKE BACTERIUM

S♀ NONE IN 80% OF CASES; OTHERS MAY HAVE VAGINAL DISCHARGE OR PAIN OR BLEEDING DURING URINATION

S♂ NONE IN 30-50% OF CASES; OTHERS MAY HAVE DISCHARGE FROM PENIS, BURNING WITH URINATION, PAIN OR SWELLING OF TESTICLES, LOW FEVER

T 7-21 DAYS

Rx CURABLE WITH ANTIBIOTICS

U♀ ABDOMINAL PAIN, BLEEDING BETWEEN PERIODS, P.I.D. (SEE BELOW), INFERTILITY

U♂ INFLAMMATION OF EPIDIDYMIS, INFERTILITY

GONORRHEA

ALSO KNOWN AS THE "CLAP" FOR SOME REASON.

O NESSERIA GONORRHOEAE, A BACTERIUM

S♀ NO SYMPTOMS IN 50-80% OF CASES; OTHERS SIMILAR TO CHLAMYDIA

S♂ ITCHING, BURNING, OR PAIN WITH URINATION; DISCHARGE FROM PENIS

T 2 DAYS - 3 WEEKS

Rx CURABLE WITH ANTIBIOTICS, EXCEPT FOR SOME RESISTANT STRAINS

U♀ P.I.D. (SEE BELOW), INFERTILITY, MAY BE PASSED TO NEWBORNS DURING CHILDBIRTH

U♂ ABCESSES IN PROSTATE, INFECTION OF EPIDIDYMIS, INFERTILITY

P.I.D. (PELVIC INFLAMMATORY DISEASE)

O UNTREATED CHLAMYDIA OR GONORRHEA MAY LEAD TO P.I.D.

S♀ PAIN IN LOWER ABDOMEN, BLEEDING BETWEEN PERIODS, PERSISTENT FEVER

T WEEKS TO MONTHS

Rx ANTIBIOTICS, SURGERY

U♀ INFERTILITY, ARTHRITIS, OTHER CHRONIC PROBLEMS

THIS ONE JUST HURTS LIKE HELL!

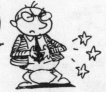

SYPHILIS

O TREPONEMA PALLIDUM, A BACTERIUM

S PRIMARY (EARLY) STAGE: RED, PAINLESS SORE (CHANCRE) ON GENITALS AT SITE OF BACTERIAL ENTRY; SECONDARY STAGE: SKIN RASH OVER BODY, INCLUDING PALMS OF HANDS AND SOLES OF FEET

T PRIMARY: 1-2 WEEKS; SECONDARY: 6 WEEKS - 6 MONTHS AFTER CHANCRE APPEARED

Rx CURABLE WITH ANTIBIOTICS

U THE TERTIARY, OR ADVANCED, STAGE, BRINGS ULCERS OF INTERNAL ORGANS, INCLUDING THE BRAIN, EYE PROBLEMS, NEUROLOGICAL DISORDERS, AND MENTAL DISTURBANCE

NOTE: THESE 4 ARE CAUSED BY BACTERIA AND CAN BE EASILY TREATED IF CAUGHT EARLY.

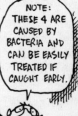

VAGINAL INFECTIONS

EVEN WHEN HEALTHY, THE VAGINA PLAYS HOST TO BILLIONS OF HARMLESS BACTERIA. OCCASIONALLY, SOMETHING UPSETS THE NORMAL BACTERIAL MIX, AND A BACTERIAL INFECTION RESULTS.

POSSIBLE CAUSES INCLUDE SEXUAL CONTACT, STRESS, CONTRACEPTIVE HORMONES, ANTIBIOTICS, DOUCHING, EVEN SYNTHETIC UNDERWEAR (HOTTER THAN COTTON!). VAGINAL INFECTIONS ARE VERY COMMON, AFFECTING 3 OUT OF 4 WOMEN AT ONE TIME OR ANOTHER.

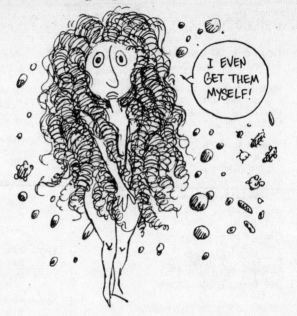

MEN CAN ALSO CARRY THE ORGANISMS THAT CAUSE VAGINAL INFECTIONS AND MAY SOMETIMES HAVE SYMPTOMS TOO.

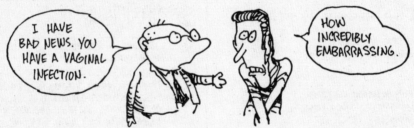

FOR BOTH SEXES, SYMPTOMS, WHEN THEY OCCUR, COME 2-21 DAYS AFTER EXPOSURE. THE MAIN CONSEQUENCE IS DISCOMFORT SO EXTREME IT WILL DRIVE YOU TO THE DOCTOR SOONER OR LATER!

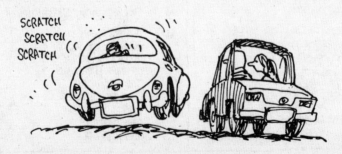

BACTERIAL VAGINOSIS

O — USUALLY GARDNERELLA VAGINALIS, A BACTERIUM

S♀ — ITCH, DISCHARGE WITH FISHY ODOR THAT IS MORE INTENSE WHEN COMBINED WITH SEMEN

S♂ — USUALLY NONE; POSSIBLE INFLAMMATION OF URETHRA OR GLANS

Rx♀ — IN MILD CASES, AN ANTIBACTERIAL DOUCHE OF POVODINE IODINE; IN MORE SERIOUS CASES, STRONGER DOUCHE OR ORAL ANTIBIOTICS

Rx♂ — ORAL ANTIBIOTICS

T,U — SEE PREVIOUS PAGE. (THE CONDITION IS SO UNCOMFORTABLE, SEEKING TREATMENT IS INEVITABLE.)

YEAST INFECTION
(CANDIDIASIS)

O — CANDIDA ALBICANS, A FUNGUS THAT LIVES NORMALLY IN THE VAGINAS OF MANY WOMEN BUT IS USUALLY CONTROLLED NATURALLY BY THE BODY.

S♀ — REDNESS AND INTENSE ITCHINESS OF VAGINA AND VULVA; COTTAGE-CHEESELIKE DISCHARGE

S♂ — USUALLY NONE

Rx — DOUCHES WITH SOLUTIONS OF VINEGAR OR YOGURT (MILD ACIDS); ANTIFUNGAL MEDICATIONS; FOR SOME WOMEN, DIET HELPS (AVOIDING SUGAR AND ALCOHOL, EATING PLENTY OF YOGURT).

T,U — SEE PREVIOUS PAGE.

TRICHOMONIASIS
("TRICK")

O — TRICHOMONAS VAGINALIS

S♀ — INTENSE ITCHINESS; FROTHY, BAD-SMELLING DISCHARGE; PAIN DURING INTERCOURSE

S♂ — USUALLY NONE; POSSIBLE PAINFUL URINATION

Rx — ORAL METRONIDAZOLE OR OTHER MEDICATION; BOTH PARTNERS MUST BE TREATED TO AVOID REINFECTION.

T,U — SEE PREVIOUS PAGE.

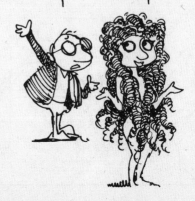

OH, MOTHER NATURE, HOW CAN YOU **DO** THIS TO PEOPLE?

WELL... BACTERIA AND YEAST ARE MY "CHILDREN" TOO...

URINARY TRACT INFECTIONS (UTIs)

CAN ALSO BE CAUSED BY SEXUAL ACTIVITY... BOTH WOMEN AND MEN CAN GET THEM... AND AN ASSORTMENT OF ORGANISMS CAN CAUSE THEM.

- **O**   VARIOUS, INCLUDING CHLAMYDIA, N. GONORRHOEAE, UREAPLASMA, UREALYTICUM, AND E. COLI
- **T**   DAYS TO WEEKS
- **S♀**   MAY BE NONE, BUT SEE CYSTITIS BELOW; POSSIBLE ITCHING AND BURNING WITH URINATION
- **S♂**   PAINFUL, FREQUENT URINATION, ITCH AFTER URINATION, WHITE OR YELLOW DISCHARGE FROM PENIS
- **Rx**   CURABLE WITH ANTIBIOTICS   **U** POSSIBLE INFERTILITY

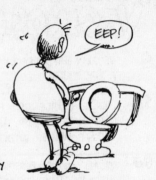

EEP!

CYSTITIS, ALSO KNOWN AS BLADDER INFECTION OR "HONEYMOON CYSTITIS," AFFECTS

ONLY WOMEN, WHO CAN NOT PASS IT TO MEN. IT HAPPENS WHEN EXCESSIVE FRICTION DAMAGES THE REGION AROUND THE URETHRA, ALLOWING BACTERIA TO ENTER THE URINARY TRACT.

- **O**   USUALLY E. COLI   **T** HOURS TO DAYS
- **S♀**   PAIN, BURNING, FREQUENT URINATION
- **Rx**   DRINK PLENTY OF WATER; DRINK CRANBERRY JUICE; APPLY WARM WATER TO URETHRA WHILE URINATING; ORAL ANTIBIOTICS
- **U♀**   POSSIBLE KIDNEY INFECTION, FEVER

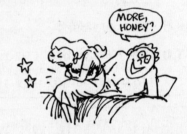

MORE, HONEY?

TO PREVENT CYSTITIS BEFORE IT STARTS:

1 DRINK PLENTY OF LIQUIDS, ESPECIALLY BEFORE AND AFTER SEX. KEEP EVERYTHING FLOWING IN THE RIGHT DIRECTION.

2 USE A LUBRICANT DURING INTERCOURSE TO PROTECT DELICATE TISSUE.

3 IF YOU USE A DIAPHRAGM AND GET FREQUENT UTIs, HAVE THE SIZE CHECKED. IT MAY BE PRESSING ON YOUR BLADDER, CAUSING STRESS.

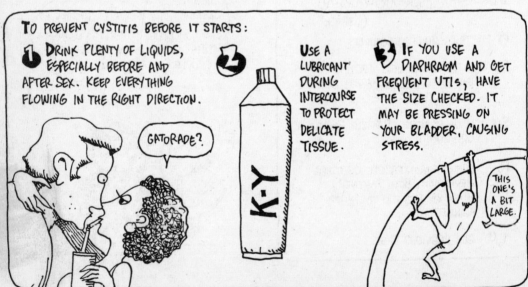

GATORADE?

K-Y

THIS ONE'S A BIT LARGE.

PARASITES

ARE NOT DISEASES EXACTLY, BUT LITTLE ANIMALS. THEY'RE MORE OF AN ANNOYING NUISANCE THAN A SERIOUS HEALTH THREAT. ASIDE FROM FLEAS, THERE ARE TWO WORTH MENTIONING.

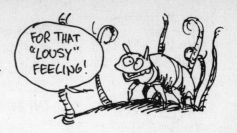

"FOR THAT "LOUSY" FEELING!"

PUBIC LICE, or "CRABS"

ARE LITTLE, BITING BUGS THAT ATTACH THEIR EGGS ("NITS") TO PUBIC HAIR.

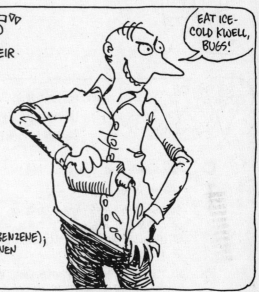

EAT ICE-COLD KWELL, BUGS!

O THE CRAB LOUSE

T INSTANT. WITHIN A WEEK, NITS BEGIN TO HATCH

S ITCH. CRAWLING SENSATION. VISIBLE LICE AND NITS. (NITS LOOK LIKE DANDRUFF, BUT ARE ROUND AND ATTACHED TO THE HAIR STALK.)

Rx OVER-THE-COUNTER LOTIONS (NIX, RID); PRESCRIPTION LOTIONS (KWELL, GAMMA-BENZENE); WASH ALL CLOTHES, TOWELS, AND BED LINEN AND DRY THEM ON HIGH SETTING

SCABIES ARE SMALLER AND FEEL WORSE THAN CRABS.

O SARCOPTES SCABIEI, A NEARLY INVISIBLE MITE

T A FEW DAYS

S RED, VERY ITCHY RASH, WHICH MAY BE ON GENITALS, BUTTOCKS, FEET, WRISTS, ABDOMEN, ARMPITS, AND SCALP.

Rx PRESCRIPTION LOTION, USUALLY CONTAINING LINDANE. (CAUTION: LINDANE IS TOXIC TO CHILDREN.) AS WITH LICE, WASH EVERYTHING.

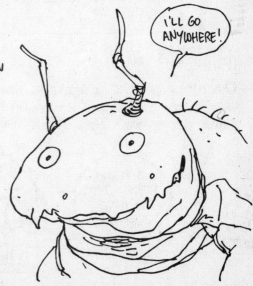

I'LL GO ANYWHERE!

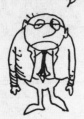

NOW SOME MORE DISCOURAGING ONES...

NOW WE COME TO FOUR STDs FOR WHICH MODERN MEDICINE HAS NO CURE. THEY ARE CAUSED BY VIRUSES, AGAINST WHICH MEDICINE HAS MADE LITTLE PROGRESS. ONLY ONE OF THESE DISEASES, HEPATITIS, CAN BE PREVENTED BY VACCINATION.

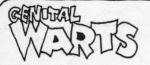 GENITAL WARTS

ALMOST SOUND RIDICULOUS, BUT THEY ARE PESKY, UNSIGHTLY, AND CAN BE WORSE THAN A NUISANCE. IN WOMEN, GENITAL WARTS INCREASE THE RISK OF CERVICAL CANCER.

O HUMAN PAPILLOMA VIRUS

T 1-6 MONTHS

S BUMPS OF VARYING APPEARANCE ON OR AROUND GENITALS, INCLUDING INTERNALLY. NOT GENERALLY PAINFUL OR ITCHY.

R$_x$ USUALLY DOCTORS DO NOTHING, SINCE WARTS USUALLY RETURN. IN EXTREME CASES, THEY ARE REMOVED SURGICALLY OR TREATED WITH CHEMICALS.

U VIRUS REMAINS IN BODY EVEN IF WARTS ARE REMOVED. RECURRENCES MAY EVENTUALLY STOP.

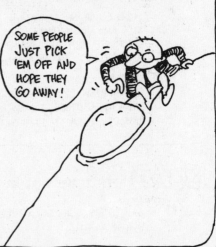

SOME PEOPLE JUST PICK 'EM OFF AND HOPE THEY GO AWAY!

HERPES

ONE OUT OF SIX OR SEVEN AMERICANS NOW CARRIES THE HERPES VIRUS, BUT JUST BECAUSE IT'S COMMON DOES NOT MEAN IT ISN'T SERIOUS. HERPES SORES CAN BE AN AVENUE THROUGH WHICH MORE SERIOUS VIRUSES, LIKE H.I.V., CAN ENTER THE BODY.

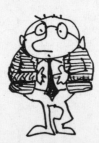

IT'S REALLY BETTER NOT TO HAVE HERPES!

HERPES (CONT'D.)

O HERPES SIMPLEX VIRUS 2 (HSV 2); SIMILAR TO HSV 1, WHICH CAUSES "COLD SORES" AROUND THE MOUTH. THROUGH ORAL SEX, EITHER HERPES VIRUS CAN INFECT EITHER PLACE.

T 3-20 DAYS

S AT THE FIRST OUTBREAK, HERPES CAN PRODUCE FLU-LIKE SYMPTOMS: FEVER, CHILLS, AND SWOLLEN LYMPH NODES. AT THE SAME TIME, SMALL ITCHY BUMPS APPEAR ON THE GENITALS. BUMPS TURN TO BLISTERS, WHICH FINALLY BURST. LATER OUTBREAKS RAISE BLISTERS WITHOUT FEVER, ETC. SERIOUS EYE INFECTIONS ARE ALSO POSSIBLE.

R$_x$ NOTHING FOOLPROOF. ACYCLOVIR, ORAL OR TOPICAL, MAY REDUCE SYMPTOMS OR DETER OUTBREAKS. SOME PEOPLE USE ICEPACKS, BAKING SODA, OR L-LYSINE. CERTAIN FOODS (NUTS, CITRUS), MAY TRIGGER OUTBREAKS, IN WHICH CASE AVOID THEM. LOOSE PANTS AND COTTON UNDERWEAR ARE EASIER ON THE REGION TOO.

U SAME RESULTS, TREATED OR UNTREATED. OUTBREAKS TEND TO BE MILDER AND LESS FREQUENT OVER TIME. SOME PEOPLE NEVER HAVE SYMPTOMS AFTER THE FIRST OUTBREAK. THE VIRUS, HOWEVER, STILL LURKS IN THE NERVOUS SYSTEM, AND BLISTERS MAY RECUR DURING TIMES OF STRESS.

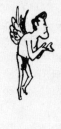
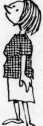

THE ONSET OF HERPES CAN BE DEVASTATING.

YES. IT PUT ME OFF SEX FOR DAYS.

HERPES CAN SPREAD EVEN WHEN THERE ARE NO ACTIVE LESIONS. IF YOU HAVE THIS STD, BE CONSIDERATE OF YOURSELF AND OTHERS.

☆ WASH HANDS OFTEN.

☆ KEEP HANDS OUT OF EYES DURING OUTBREAKS.

☆ SIT ON A TOWEL AT SAUNAS AND POOLS!

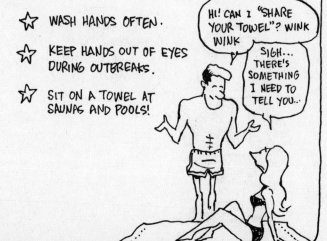

HI! CAN I "SHARE YOUR TOWEL"? WINK WINK

SIGH... THERE'S SOMETHING I NEED TO TELL YOU...

WARNING:

HERPES CAN BLIND NEWBORN BABIES. PREGNANT WOMEN AND THEIR PARTNERS SHOULD DISCUSS APPROPRIATE PRECAUTIONS WITH THEIR MEDICAL PRACTITIONER IF THEY HAVE BEEN EXPOSED TO HERPES.

HEPATITIS,

A VERY SERIOUS INFECTION OF THE LIVER, CAN BE TRANSMITTED IN VARIOUS WAYS. ONE STRAIN, HEPATITIS **A**, IS SPREAD VIA FECES, AS FROM ANUS TO MOUTH, OR ANUS TO FINGER TO MOUTH. HEPATITIS **B**, WHICH IS USUALLY MORE SEVERE, PASSES VIA BLOOD, SEMEN, VAGINAL SECRETIONS, SALIVA, AND URINE. UNFORTUNATELY, THIS MAKES HEPATITIS B THE KIND MOST OFTEN TRANSMITTED SEXUALLY.

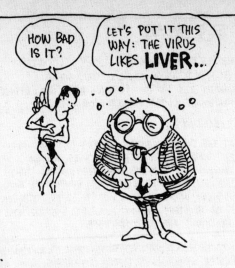

O   HEPATITIS VIRUS (A OR B)   **T** 1-4 MONTHS

S   SEVERAL WEEKS OF FEVER, FATIGUE, QUEASINESS, ABDOMINAL PAIN, JAUNDICE (YELLOWING OF SKIN IN WHITE PEOPLE, YELLOWING OF EYES IN OTHERS), URINE THE COLOR OF DARK TEA

R   NO MEDICAL CURE, EXCEPT TO WAIT IT OUT. REST AND PLENTY OF FLUIDS.

U   POSSIBLE PERMANENT LIVER DAMAGE; CAN BE FATAL

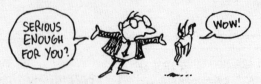

THERE IS A VACCINE AGAINST HEPATITIS B. VACCINATION IS A GOOD IDEA FOR PEOPLE WITH MULTIPLE SEX PARTNERS.

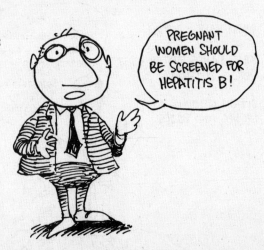

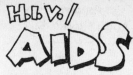

HIV/ AIDS (Aquired Immune Deficiency Syndrome)

The deadliest STD, AIDS attacks the body's immune system, reducing its ability to fight off all other infections. As far as we know, AIDS is a new disease, first infecting human populations in the 1950s and spreading rapidly only after around 1980. Because the disease is so new, AIDS research and treatment are evolving rapidly. **HIV**, the virus responsible for AIDS, can be passed via blood, semen, vaginal secretions, and breast milk.

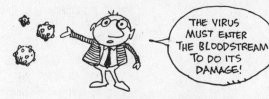

THE VIRUS MUST ENTER THE BLOODSTREAM TO DO ITS DAMAGE!

O HUMAN IMMUNODEFICIENCY VIRUS (H.I.V.)

T SEVERAL MONTHS TO 10 YEARS

S FLU-LIKE SYMPTOMS OR NO SYMPTOMS IN EARLY STAGES OF INFECTION. LATER COME WEIGHT LOSS, PERSISTENT FEVER, NIGHT SWEATS, DIARRHEA, SWOLLEN LYMPH NODES, A BRUISELIKE RASH, AND NAGGING COUGH. AIDS PATIENTS ALSO FALL PREY TO "OPPORTUNISTIC" INFECTIONS, ESPECIALLY CERTAIN TYPES OF PNEUMONIA, TUBERCULOSIS, AND CANCER. IN THE LATER STAGES, MENTAL PROBLEMS ("AIDS DEMENTIA") MAY DEVELOP.

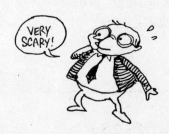

VERY SCARY!

Rx A CHANGING ARRAY OF MEDICATIONS; OPPORTUNISTIC INFECTIONS ARE TREATED WITH ANTIBIOTICS. AZT RETARDS THE DISEASE; SOME NEW (AND EXPENSIVE) COMBINATIONS OF PROTEASE INHIBITORS ARE HIGHLY SUCCESSFUL IN SOME PATIENTS, LESS SO IN OTHERS. GOOD HEALTH PRACTICES CAN DELAY THE ONSET OF SYMPTOMS OR REDUCE THEIR SEVERITY.

U AIDS IS INCURABLE. A FEW PEOPLE — LESS THAN 1% OF THE POPULATION — APPEAR TO BE IMMUNE. FOR THE REST, THE IMMUNE SYSTEM EVENTUALLY COLLAPSES, AND THE PATIENT DIES FROM A COMBINATION OF FACTORS.

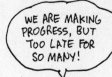

WE ARE MAKING PROGRESS, BUT TOO LATE FOR SO MANY!

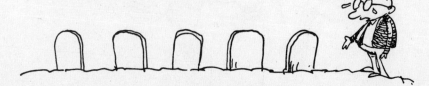

AIDS IS SCARY... SO SCARY THAT SOME PEOPLE REFUSE TO FACE THE POSSIBILITY OF CATCHING IT... COMBINE THAT WITH THE FACT THAT, IN THE U.S., THE EPIDEMIC BEGAN IN THE GAY MALE POPULATION AND SPREAD TO PEOPLE WHO SHARE NEEDLES TO SHOOT DRUGS, AND YOU GET SOME UNFORTUNATE

MYTHS ABOUT AIDS.

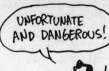

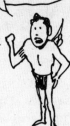

MYTH:

YOU DON'T HAVE TO WORRY IF YOU'RE NOT IN A SO-CALLED HIGH-RISK GROUP (I.E., GAY MEN OR INTRAVENOUS DRUG USERS).

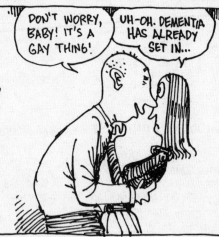

REALITY:

THE RISK OF AIDS IS REAL. EVEN THOUGH THE ABSOLUTE NUMBER OF CASES IS STILL HIGHEST IN HIGH-RISK POPULATIONS, THE RATE OF INCREASE IS NOW HIGH AMONG HETEROSEXUALS, ESPECIALLY WOMEN AND MINORITIES.

MYTH:

AIDS IS A CONSPIRACY AGAINST BLACKS AND/OR GAYS. THE VIRUS WAS DEVELOPED IN A GOVERNMENT LAB FOR BIOLOGICAL WARFARE.

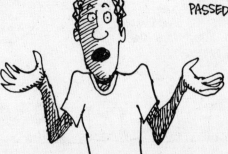

REALITY:

ALL SCIENTIFIC EVIDENCE POINTS TO H.I.V.'s ORIGIN IN AFRICA. IT APPEARS TO BE A MUTANT FORM OF A MONKEY VIRUS THAT SOMEHOW PASSED TO HUMANS.

MYTH:

(THE STRANGE FLIP SIDE OF MYTH #1): H.I.V. IS EASY TO "CATCH." YOU SHOULDN'T TOUCH OR KISS ANYONE WITH AIDS.

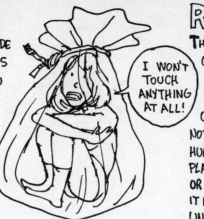

I WON'T TOUCH ANYTHING AT ALL!

REALITY:

THE VIRUS IS FRAGILE. IT DIES QUICKLY OUTSIDE THE BODY AND WHEN EXPOSED TO SPERMICIDES, BLEACH (FOR NEEDLES), AND OTHER DISINFECTANTS. YOU CAN NOT GET AIDS FROM SHAKING HANDS, HUGGING, NON-SLOBBERY KISSING, PLAYING SPORTS, DONATING BLOOD, OR BEING BITTEN BY MOSQUITOES. IT IS NOT TRANSMITTED BY SALIVA, UNLESS THERE IS BLOOD IN IT, NOR BY TEARS, SWEAT, WATER, SWIMMING POOLS, OR HOT TUBS.

TO REPEAT:

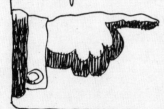

HIV CAN ONLY BE PASSED WHEN INFECTED BLOOD, SEMEN, VAGINAL SECRETIONS, OR BREAST MILK HAVE A DIRECT PATHWAY TO THE BLOODSTREAM. THE RAPID SPREAD OF THE DISEASE IS A RESULT OF PEOPLE HAVING RISKY, UNPROTECTED SEX WITH MANY PARTNERS.

MYTH:

CONDOMS DO NOT REALLY PROTECT ANYONE FROM AIDS.

REALITY:

IF USED PROPERLY, LATEX CONDOMS DRAMATICALLY REDUCE THE RISK OF INFECTION (BUT NOT TO ZERO, WE HAVE TO ADD!!).

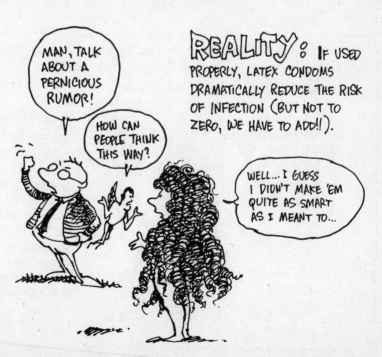

MAN, TALK ABOUT A PERNICIOUS RUMOR!

HOW CAN PEOPLE THINK THIS WAY?

WELL... I GUESS I DIDN'T MAKE 'EM QUITE AS SMART AS I MEANT TO...

THE AIDS TEST

AIDS IS SO FRIGHTENING THAT MANY PEOPLE REFUSE TO BE TESTED FOR IT, JUST TO AVOID DEALING WITH POTENTIAL BAD NEWS. STILL, IF YOU THINK YOU MAY HAVE BEEN EXPOSED TO H.I.V., THERE ARE GOOD REASONS FOR TAKING THE TEST.

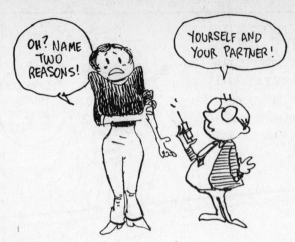

FOR ONE THING, THE VAST MAJORITY OF H.I.V. TESTS TURN UP "NEGATIVE" RESULTS — I.E., NO INFECTION. (THIS IS NOT AN EXCUSE FOR RISKY BEHAVIOR!)

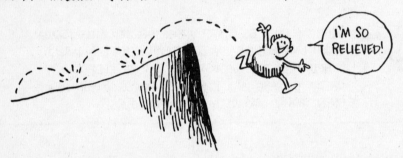

EVEN A "POSITIVE" RESULT MUST BE CONFIRMED BY A SECOND TEST BEFORE A DEFINITE DIAGNOSIS CAN BE MADE. IF THE RESULT IS FINALLY ONE OF H.I.V.-POSITIVE, TREATMENT SHOULD BEGIN AS EARLY AS POSSIBLE, AND SOME IMPORTANT CONVERSATIONS NEED TO HAPPEN.

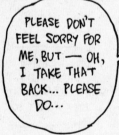

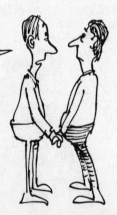

SCIENTIFIC NOTE: THE MOST COMMONLY USED H.I.V. TEST LOOKS NOT FOR VIRUS BUT FOR VIRAL ANTIBODIES. THESE ARE CELLS PRODUCED BY THE IMMUNE SYSTEM AND TARGETED AT H.I.V. SINCE IT CAN TAKE 2 TO 6 MONTHS TO BUILD UP A DETECTABLE LEVEL OF ANTIBODIES, THE TEST MAY NOT REVEAL AN INFECTION IN ITS EARLY PHASE. ANYONE WHO SUSPECTS RECENT H.I.V. EXPOSURE SHOULD REPEAT THE TEST AFTER 6 MONTHS.

STAYING HEALTHY

IF STDs ARE SO UNPLEASANT, WHY DOESN'T EVERYONE TAKE PRECAUTIONS AGAINST THEM? WHEN IT COMES TO SEX, PEOPLE ARE REALLY BRILLIANT AT INVENTING STUPID EXCUSES FOR NOT TAKING CARE OF THEMSELVES!

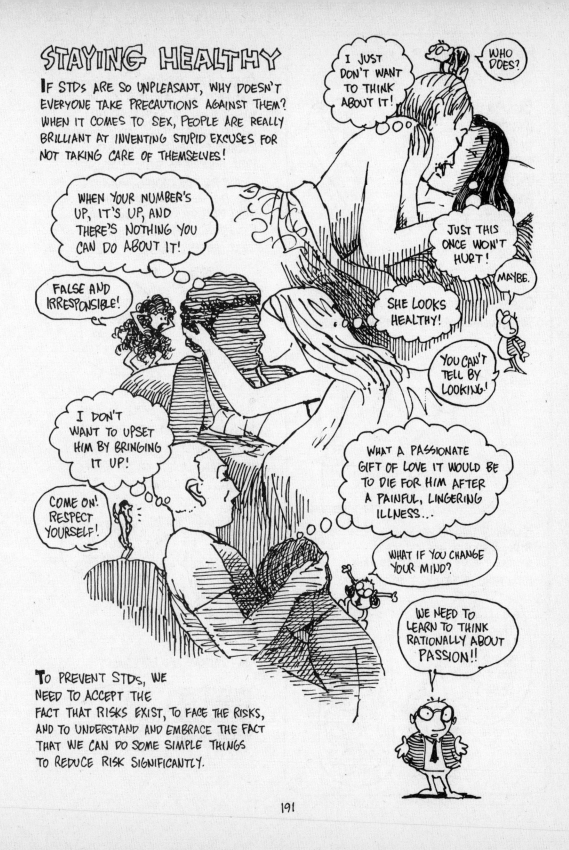

TO PREVENT STDs, WE NEED TO ACCEPT THE FACT THAT RISKS EXIST, TO FACE THE RISKS, AND TO UNDERSTAND AND EMBRACE THE FACT THAT WE CAN DO SOME SIMPLE THINGS TO REDUCE RISK SIGNIFICANTLY.

HERE ARE A FEW SIMPLE HEALTH ENHANCERS:

GOOD GENITAL HYGIENE — I.E., WASHING — ESPECIALLY UNDER THE FORESKIN FOR UNCIRCUMCISED MALES.

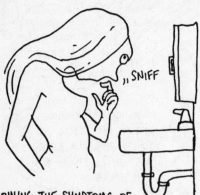

CHECKING OURSELVES AND OUR PARTNERS FOR GENITAL SORES OR UNUSUAL DISCHARGES.

,, SNIFF

KNOWING THE SYMPTOMS OF STDs; SEEKING MEDICAL CARE AT THE ONSET OF SYMPTOMS; AND FOLLOWING TREATMENT INSTRUCTIONS.

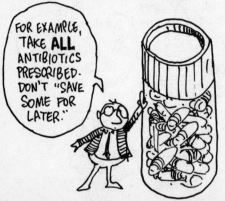

FOR EXAMPLE, TAKE **ALL** ANTIBIOTICS PRESCRIBED— DON'T "SAVE SOME FOR LATER."

AND (VERY IMPORTANT): INFORMING OUR PARTNERS ABOUT STDs WE MIGHT HAVE OR SYMPTOMS THAT MIGHT INDICATE ONE; ANY POSSIBLE RECENT EXPOSURE TO AN STD; PAST HISTORY OF STDs; CURRENT LIFESTYLE, INCLUDING MULTIPLE SEX PARTNERS OR INJECTION-DRUG USE; OR HISTORY OF SAME; AND H.I.V. STATUS AS DETERMINED BY TEST, NOT BY GUESS.

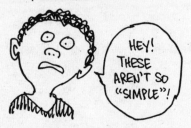

HEY! THESE AREN'T SO "SIMPLE"!

AS WE SAID IN CHAPTER 6, THIS REQUIRES SOME FAITH THAT YOUR PARTNER WILL APPRECIATE HONESTY MORE THAN DECEPTION OR WITHHOLDING OF INFORMATION.

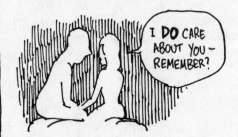

I **DO** CARE ABOUT YOU— REMEMBER?

AND, FINALLY AND ESPECIALLY:

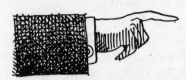

SAFER SEX PRACTICES

(WE SAY "SAFER" RATHER THAN "SAFE," SINCE EVERY SEXUAL ACT CARRIES SOME RISK THESE DAYS. 100% SAFE SEX CAN ONLY HAPPEN BETWEEN TWO TOTALLY TRUSTWORTHY, MONOGAMOUS, UNINFECTED PARTNERS.)

 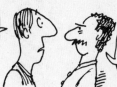

HOW DO I KNOW THAT'S YOU?

DON'T YOU TRUST ME WHEN I SAY YOU CAN TRUST ME?

WELL, NO SEX AT ALL IS NEARLY 100% SAFE... AND SO IS MASTURBATION...

HEALTHY, BUT LONELY...

WITH ANOTHER PERSON, THE SAFEST THINGS ARE HUGGING, KISSING (IF THERE'S NO BLOOD IN THE SALIVA), PETTING, MANUAL SEX (UNLESS THERE ARE SORES OR ABRASIONS ON HANDS OR GENITALS), AND SEX TOYS (WASHED BETWEEN USES).

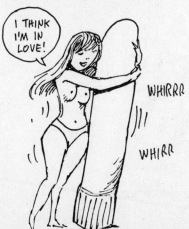

I THINK I'M IN LOVE!

WHIRRR

WHIRR

A LITTLE RISKIER, BUT STILL CONSIDERED SAFE:

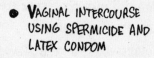

- VAGINAL INTERCOURSE USING SPERMICIDE AND LATEX CONDOM

- FELLATIO WITH CONDOM

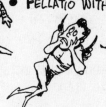

NOBODY'S FAVORITE, BUT TRY MINT-FLAVORED!

- CUNNILINGUS IF THE WOMAN IS NOT MENSTRUATING AND HAS NO VAGINAL INFECTION. (USE A LATEX DENTAL DAM FOR ADDED PROTECTION.)

- ANAL INTERCOURSE — MAYBE — WITH A CONDOM AND SPERMICIDE. (SINCE ANAL INTERCOURSE IS THE RISKIEST KIND OF ALL, CONDOM FAILURE IS BAD NEWS HERE.)

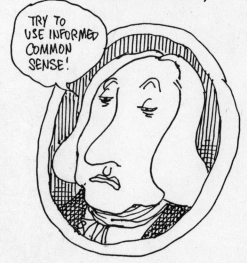

TRY TO USE INFORMED COMMON SENSE!

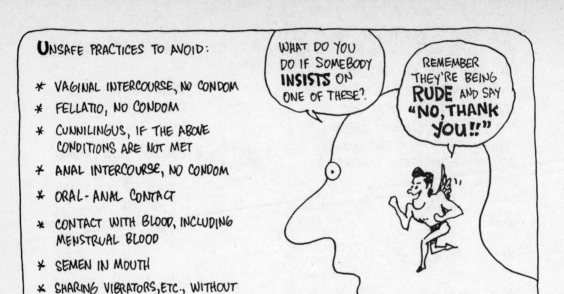

So... GO FORTH... TAKE CARE... GOOD LUCK... AND REMEMBER: IF YOU DON'T DISCUSS STDs, AND YOU DON'T PRACTICE SAFER SEX, YOU AND YOUR PARTNER HAVE SILENTLY "AGREED" THAT THIS SUBJECT IS NOT IMPORTANT, AND UNSAFE SEX IS O.K.

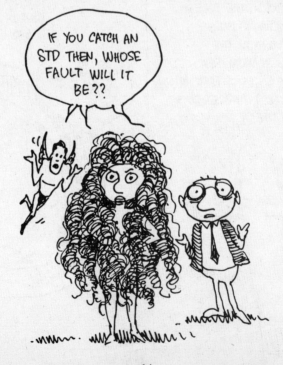

· CHAPTER 11 ·
UNINVITED SEX

T IS NEITHER LEGAL
NOR POLITE TO PERFORM
SEX ACTS WITH AN
UNWILLING PARTNER.
IN THIS CHAPTER, WE
FOCUS ON VARIOUS
KINDS OF SEXUAL
BEHAVIOR THAT CAN
WIN YOU A DATE
WITH THE AUTHORITIES.

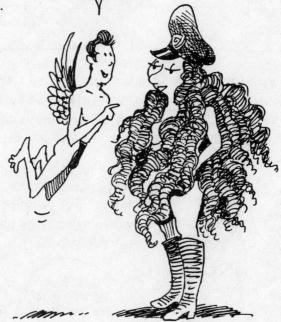

HEY!
ARRESTING
OUTFIT!

LET'S START WITH THE HEAVY STUFF...

RAPE IS FORCED SEX THAT INVOLVES PENILE-
VAGINAL PENETRATION. AMONG SOME ANIMALS,
EVERY SEX ACT LOOKS LIKE RAPE. THE MALE HOUSE
FLY, FOR INSTANCE, REPEATEDLY JUMPS THE FEMALE,
WHILE SHE KEEPS TRYING TO THROW HIM OFF.

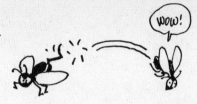

WOW!

FOR HUMANS, A
MORE VERBAL SPECIES
CAPABLE OF ASKING
FOR WHAT WE WANT
(OR DON'T WANT),

RAPE IS THE ULTIMATE
SEXUAL VIOLATION, A
DENIAL OF FEMALE
CHOICE, A GENETIC
HIJACKING, AND A
PHYSICAL ASSAULT.

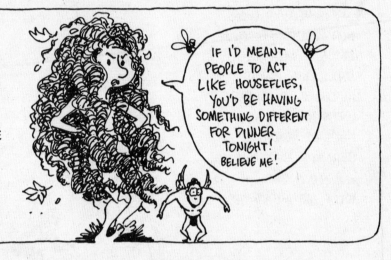

IF I'D MEANT
PEOPLE TO ACT
LIKE HOUSEFLIES,
YOU'D BE HAVING
SOMETHING DIFFERENT
FOR DINNER
TONIGHT!
BELIEVE ME!

IN THE OLD, MALE-CENTERED VIEW OF THINGS, RAPE VIOLATED A WOMAN'S HONOR AND SO
REDUCED HER VALUE TO HER MALE PROTECTORS (FATHER OR HUSBAND). IN OTHER WORDS,
RAPE WAS CONSIDERED A CRIME AGAINST **MEN!** SO RAPISTS WERE PUNISHED HARSHLY,
AND THE DISHONORED WOMAN MIGHT BE ILL-TREATED AS WELL.

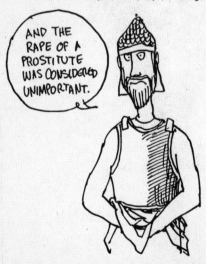

AND THE
RAPE OF A
PROSTITUTE
WAS CONSIDERED
UNIMPORTANT.

WITH THE RISE OF FEMINISM, RAPE WAS
REEVALUATED. WOMEN URGED SYMPATHY,
RATHER THAN DISHONOR, FOR THE VICTIM.
AND OF COURSE THEY HAVE LITTLE USE FOR
THE PERPETRATOR.

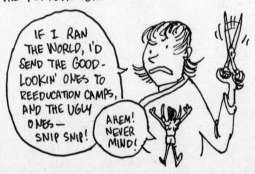

IF I RAN
THE WORLD, I'D
SEND THE GOOD-
LOOKIN' ONES TO
REEDUCATION CAMPS,
AND THE UGLY
ONES —
SNIP SNIP!

AHEM!
NEVER
MIND!

We tend to imagine rapists as psychopaths who lurk in the bushes, ready to pounce. This is a myth, not entirely false, but not entirely true, either. Psychological tests show rapists to be very similar to other men, except that rapists tend to have more trouble handling their hostile emotions.

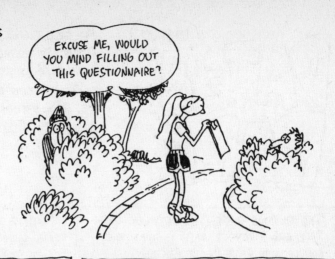

A more typical rape scenario begins with a chance meeting... it might be at school, a party, café, health club, bus stop, etc...

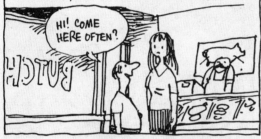

The man seems normal, friendly, even protective. The woman lets her guard down.

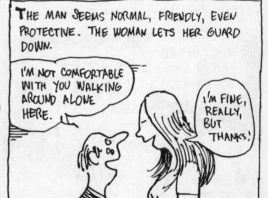

He casually maneuvers the woman into an isolated place...

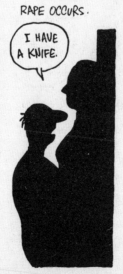

...where the rape occurs.

Weapons are involved in only about 1/3 of all rapes by strangers. At other times, a weapon may be threatened, or sheer brute force is enough.

197

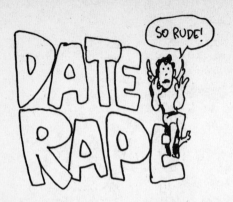

An even bigger myth than the bush-lurking psychopath is the idea that most rapes are committed by strangers. In fact, it is more common for women to be forced into sex by a dating partner, an experience shared by more than 15% of all women.

The obvious difference between date rape and stranger rape is that the couple may have "gone partway" beforehand. This can lead to confusion!

Further clouding the issue are alcohol and drugs. Most date rapes happen when one or both parties are under the influence.

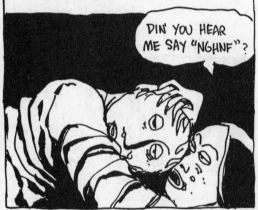

Some people say that no gentleman would take advantage of an intoxicated female.

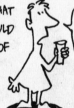

Others suggest that it's foolish to expect a drunken male to behave like a gentleman — and besides, a woman should take responsibility for her own drug use and drinking.

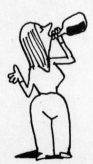

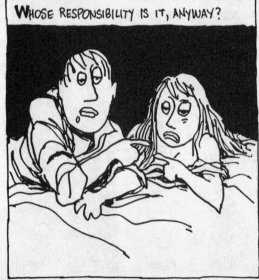

WE THINK ALL PARTIES
SHOULD TAKE RESPONSIBILITY
FOR THEIR OWN ACTIONS,
BEGINNING WITH SOME PRUDENCE
IN THE USE OF ALCOHOL AND DRUGS.

AND, GUYS, IT REALLY ISN'T O.K. TO MESS SOMEONE UP SO YOU CAN TAKE ADVANTAGE OF HER. SEX ISN'T SO GREAT WHEN ONE PARTY CAN BARELY MOVE, ANYWAY, AND BESIDES, ANY ACT OF FORCIBLE SEX IS STILL RAPE. IT CAN LAND YOU IN JAIL!

REMEMBER, WOMEN AND MEN: DRUGS IMPAIR JUDGMENT! PEOPLE UNDER THE INFLUENCE DO THINGS THEY COME TO REGRET LATER, LIKE PASSING OUT, TURNING VIOLENT, GETTING PREGNANT, CATCHING A DISEASE, ETC...

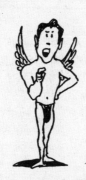

FINALLY, WHAT ABOUT THE RISK OF FALSE ACCUSATION? DATE RAPE IS A CRIME WITHOUT WITNESSES, AND GUYS FEAR VIGILANTE JUSTICE ON CAMPUS.

"NOW MAY I TOUCH YOUR INNER THIGHS?" "YES." "NOW MAY I RHYTHMICALLY PALPATE YOUR CLITORIS WITH MY INDEX FINGER?" "NHHH..."

WHOA! I MADE A TAPE RECORDING! THIS PROVES WE FOLLOWED THE UNIVERSITY PERMISSION CODE!

AMBIGUOUS RESPONSE!!

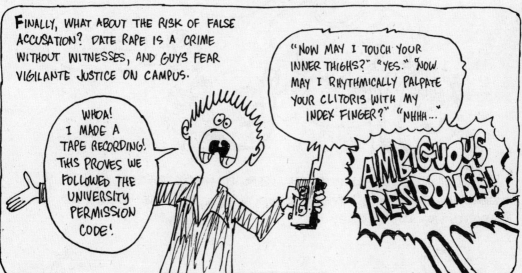

THIS IS SOMETHING OF A MYTH. ALTHOUGH WOMEN DO SOMETIMES "CRY RAPE" FOR REVENGE, FALSE ACCUSATIONS OF RAPE ARE LESS COMMON THAN FALSE REPORTS OF MOST OTHER CRIMES.

BUT VIGILANTE "JUSTICE" IS ALWAYS RUDE!

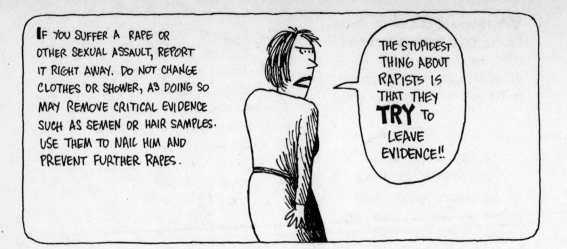

IF YOU SUFFER A RAPE OR OTHER SEXUAL ASSAULT, REPORT IT RIGHT AWAY. DO NOT CHANGE CLOTHES OR SHOWER, AS DOING SO MAY REMOVE CRITICAL EVIDENCE SUCH AS SEMEN OR HAIR SAMPLES. USE THEM TO NAIL HIM AND PREVENT FURTHER RAPES.

THE STUPIDEST THING ABOUT RAPISTS IS THAT THEY **TRY** TO LEAVE EVIDENCE!!

MEN, TOO, ARE SEXUALLY ASSAULTED, ALMOST ALWAYS BY OTHER MEN. MALE VICTIMS ARE LESS LIKELY THAN WOMEN TO REPORT THE ASSAULT. THEY MAY BE EMBARRASSED BY THEIR FAILURE TO DEFEND THEMSELVES, OR THEY MAY FEAR REPRISAL FROM THE ASSAULTER, AS IN JAIL.

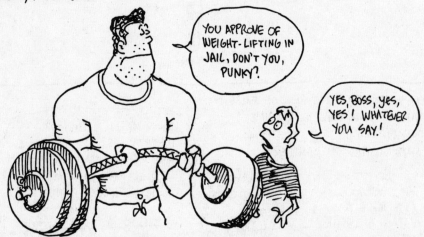

YOU APPROVE OF WEIGHT-LIFTING IN JAIL, DON'T YOU, PUNKY?

YES, BOSS, YES, YES! WHATEVER YOU SAY!

VICTIMS OF SEXUAL ASSAULT OFTEN FEEL DEPRESSED, ANXIOUS, RESTLESS, AND GUILTY. WOMEN MAY BEGIN TO LOSE DESIRE OR EVEN TO FEAR SEX. TIME, PATIENCE, AND UNDERSTANDING ARE THE CURE.

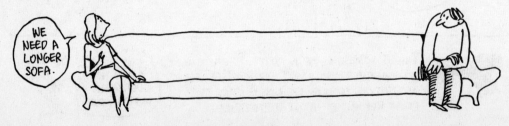

WE NEED A LONGER SOFA.

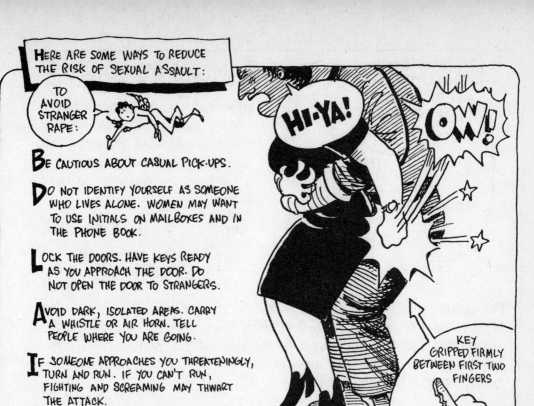

HERE ARE SOME WAYS TO REDUCE THE RISK OF SEXUAL ASSAULT:

TO AVOID STRANGER RAPE:

BE CAUTIOUS ABOUT CASUAL PICK-UPS.

DO NOT IDENTIFY YOURSELF AS SOMEONE WHO LIVES ALONE. WOMEN MAY WANT TO USE INITIALS ON MAILBOXES AND IN THE PHONE BOOK.

LOCK THE DOORS. HAVE KEYS READY AS YOU APPROACH THE DOOR. DO NOT OPEN THE DOOR TO STRANGERS.

AVOID DARK, ISOLATED AREAS. CARRY A WHISTLE OR AIR HORN. TELL PEOPLE WHERE YOU ARE GOING.

IF SOMEONE APPROACHES YOU THREATENINGLY, TURN AND RUN. IF YOU CAN'T RUN, FIGHTING AND SCREAMING MAY THWART THE ATTACK.

TAKE SELF-DEFENSE CLASSES.

HI-YA!

OW!

KEY GRIPPED FIRMLY BETWEEN FIRST TWO FINGERS

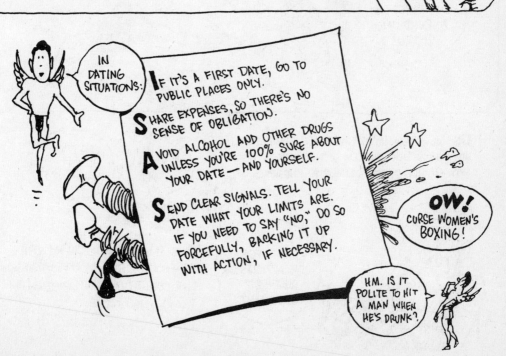

IN DATING SITUATIONS:

IF IT'S A FIRST DATE, GO TO PUBLIC PLACES ONLY.

SHARE EXPENSES, SO THERE'S NO SENSE OF OBLIGATION.

AVOID ALCOHOL AND OTHER DRUGS UNLESS YOU'RE 100% SURE ABOUT YOUR DATE — AND YOURSELF.

SEND CLEAR SIGNALS. TELL YOUR DATE WHAT YOUR LIMITS ARE. IF YOU NEED TO SAY "NO," DO SO FORCEFULLY, BACKING IT UP WITH ACTION, IF NECESSARY.

OW! CURSE WOMEN'S BOXING!

HM. IS IT POLITE TO HIT A MAN WHEN HE'S DRUNK?

201

DOES PORNOGRAPHY CAUSE RAPE?

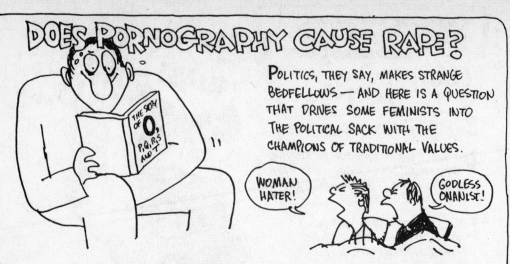

POLITICS, THEY SAY, MAKES STRANGE BEDFELLOWS — AND HERE IS A QUESTION THAT DRIVES SOME FEMINISTS INTO THE POLITICAL SACK WITH THE CHAMPIONS OF TRADITIONAL VALUES.

WOMAN HATER!

GODLESS ONANIST!

PORNOGRAPHY, ACCORDING TO ONE LINE OF FEMINIST THOUGHT, IS THE MORAL EQUIVALENT OF RAPE. SMUT REQUIRES WOMEN TO DO MEN'S BIDDING: "PORNOGRAPHY IS THE THEORY, AND RAPE IS THE PRACTICE," SAID FEMINIST ROBIN MORGAN. THE TRADITIONAL VALUES CROWD MAY NOT AGREE, BUT SINCE THEY TEND TO OPPOSE ALL PUBLIC SEXUAL EXPRESSION, THEY'RE HAPPY TO HAVE THE SUPPORT.

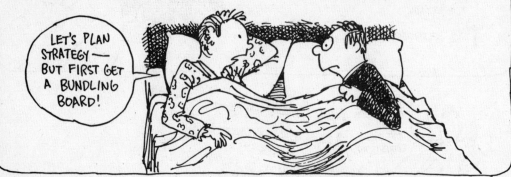

LET'S PLAN STRATEGY — BUT FIRST GET A BUNDLING BOARD!

ON THE OTHER HAND, THERE ARE FEMINISTS WHO THINK THE PROBLEM WITH SMUT IS THAT NOT ENOUGH OF IT IS AIMED AT WOMEN!

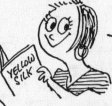

CAN'T WE CALL IT "EROTICA"?

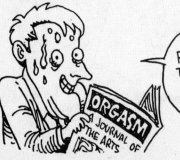

I ONLY READ IT FOR THE ARTICLES ON THE FIRST AMENDMENT!

THIS TENDS TO ALLY THEM WITH OTHER ADVOCATES OF FREE EXPRESSION, LIKE CONSTITUTIONAL LAWYERS AND PLAYBOY MAGAZINE.

SOME ARGUE THAT PORNOGRAPHY IS MAINLY FOR MASTURBATION, SO ACTUALLY IT COOLS PEOPLE DOWN.

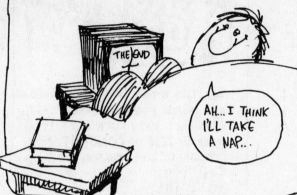

OTHERS MIGHT SAY THAT PORNOGRAPHY, BY PORTRAYING NOTHING BUT PERFECT, YIELDING FEMALES, MAY MAKE MEN RESENT REAL WOMEN, WITH THEIR HUMAN IMPERFECTIONS AND NEEDS.

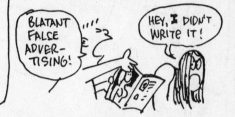

SO FAR, PSYCHOLOGICAL STUDIES SHOW LITTLE LINK BETWEEN **NON-VIOLENT** EROTICA AND SEXUAL AGGRESSION... BUT MEN EXPOSED TO **VIOLENT** SEXUAL MATERIAL DO SHOW AN INCREASE IN VIOLENT SEXUAL FANTASIES.

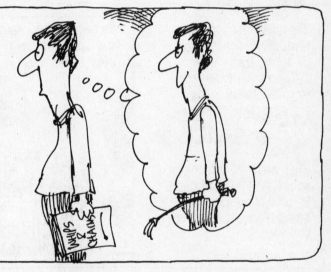

NEVERTHELESS, OVER THE PAST FEW DECADES, THE U.S. SUPREME COURT HAS (MOSTLY) PROTECTED THE RIGHTS OF PEOPLE WHO PRODUCE AND CONSUME WORKS OF ART THAT ARE TASTELESS, CRUDE, GROSS, OFFENSIVE, LEWD, AND STUPID...

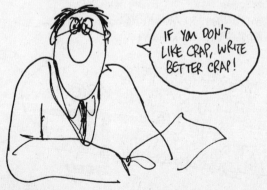

...UNLESS, THAT IS, THEY INVOLVE CHILDREN...

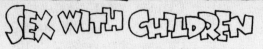

SEX WITH CHILDREN

IS ALSO UNINVITED, EVEN IF NO FORCE IS INVOLVED. A CHILD MOLESTER MAY USE BRIBES, AND MANY PEDOPHILES GO ON TO DESCRIBE THEIR RELATIONSHIPS TO BE LOVING AND MUTUAL.

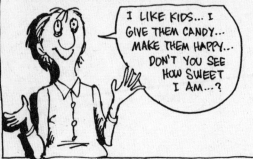

I LIKE KIDS... I GIVE THEM CANDY... MAKE THEM HAPPY... DON'T YOU SEE HOW SWEET I AM...?

SOCIETY'S ANSWER IS NOT UNREASONABLE:

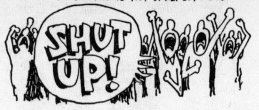

SHUT UP!

SEX, LIKE VOTING, DRINKING, AND ENTERING INTO LEGALLY BINDING AGREEMENTS, IS FOR GROWN-UPS. EVERY STATE HAS A LEGAL MINIMUM **AGE OF CONSENT.** HAVE SEX WITH SOMEONE YOUNGER, AND GO TO **JAIL.**

THE PERCENTAGE OF US WHO REPORT SOME EPISODE OF SEXUAL CONTACT IN CHILDHOOD WITH AN ADULT IS SURPRISINGLY HIGH: **25%** OF ALL WOMEN, **15%** OF ALL MEN.

(THIS INCLUDES SUCH THINGS AS INAPPROPRIATE TOUCHING BY DOCTORS OR PARENTS' FRIENDS, AS WELL AS OUT-AND-OUT RAPE.)

IS CHILD SEXUAL ABUSE ON THE RISE? IT'S HARD TO SAY. IN TIMES PAST, THERE WERE SOME THINGS ONE JUST DIDN'T TALK ABOUT.

A MAN'S HOME IS HIS CASTLE, COMPLETE WITH DUNGEON!

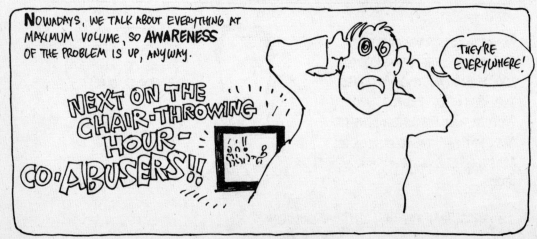

NOWADAYS, WE TALK ABOUT EVERYTHING AT MAXIMUM VOLUME, SO **AWARENESS** OF THE PROBLEM IS UP, ANYWAY.

NEXT ON THE CHAIR-THROWING HOUR— CO-ABUSERS!!

THEY'RE EVERYWHERE!

PERSISTENT SEXUAL ABUSE OF KIDS CAN DO SERIOUS HARM TO THEIR EMOTIONAL AND SEXUAL DEVELOPMENT, BUT PLEASE HEED THIS

WARNING:

THERE ARE SOME THERAPISTS WHO THINK THAT **ALL** ADULT ANXIETY, DEPRESSION, AND SEXUAL DYSFUNCTION STEM FROM SEXUAL ABUSE DURING CHILDHOOD.

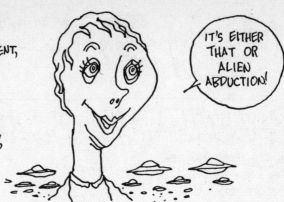

IT'S EITHER THAT OR ALIEN ABDUCTION!

IF YOU'RE FEELING BAD BUT CAN'T REMEMBER ANY SUCH THING, THESE CHARACTERS WILL TRY TO "HELP" YOU "REMEMBER" BY MAKING SUGGESTIONS DISGUISED AS QUESTIONS.

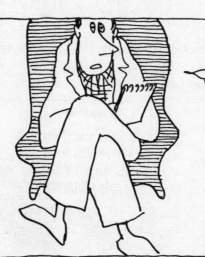

WAS YOUR FATHER HOLDING ANYTHING RESEMBLING A BANANA?

SOME FACTS ABOUT MEMORY:

1. MEMORIES OF TRAUMATIC CHILDHOOD EVENTS ARE USUALLY REMEMBERED, NOT FORGOTTEN.

2. MEMORY IS UNRELIABLE. MEMORIES CAN ERODE OR CHANGE OVER TIME.

3. FALSE "MEMORIES" CAN BE CREATED IN SUGGESTIBLE PEOPLE BY THERAPISTS, POLICE OFFICERS, OR OTHER AUTHORITY FIGURES WHOM THE "REMEMBERER" WISHES TO PLEASE.

THERAPISTS SOMETIMES TALK ABOUT "RECOVERED MEMORY," BUT IT MAY BE NO MORE THAN **IMPLANTED FANTASY.**

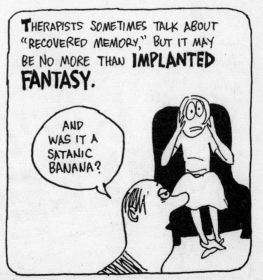

AND WAS IT A SATANIC BANANA?

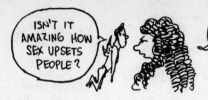

ISN'T IT AMAZING HOW SEX UPSETS PEOPLE?

YOU'RE ANNOYING ME, ELF!

SEXUAL HARASSMENT

THIRTY YEARS AGO, THE LAW KNEW NO SUCH CONCEPT. TODAY IT'S ILLEGAL. WHAT HAPPENED?

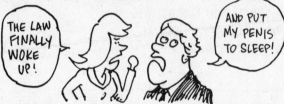

THE LAW FINALLY WOKE UP!

AND PUT MY PENIS TO SLEEP!

SEXUAL HARASSMENT MEANS PERSISTENT AND/OR UNWANTED SEXUAL ATTENTION, ESPECIALLY IN THE WORKPLACE (AND ON CAMPUS, A KIND OF WORKPLACE). THIS INCLUDES TOUCHING, FLIRTING, COMMENTS, JOKES, ETC...

SOME PEOPLE ARE NATURALLY CONCERNED ABOUT ANY LAW THAT RESTRICTS FREEDOM OF SPEECH.

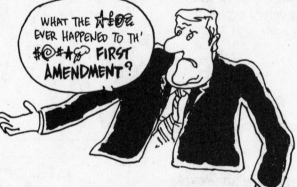

WHAT THE #±©& EVER HAPPENED TO TH' #©#& FIRST AMENDMENT?

AND THEN THERE'S THE MORE BASIC WORRY:

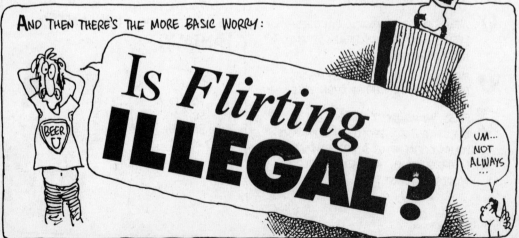

Is Flirting ILLEGAL?

UM... NOT ALWAYS...

THE SEXUAL HARASSMENT LAWS ORIGINATED IN WOMEN'S DEMANDS FOR GENDER EQUALITY IN THE WORKPLACE. WHEN FEMALES WERE FIRST HIRED TO DO TRADITIONALLY MALE JOBS, THERE WERE PLENTY OF RESENTFUL MEN — AND THEY WEREN'T BASHFUL ABOUT SAYING SO!

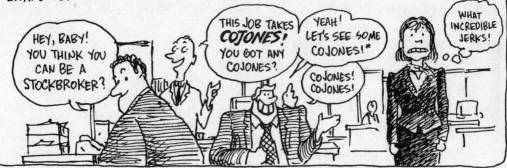

*COJONES ("KO-HO-NAYS"): SPANISH FOR "BALLS."

FOR WOMEN TO COMPETE WITH MEN, IT WAS REASONED, THEY NEEDED TO BE ABLE TO DO THEIR JOBS WITHOUT THIS KIND OF INTIMIDATION. TO PROTECT THEM FROM A HOSTILE WORKPLACE ENVIRONMENT, THE GOVERNMENT PASSED LAWS AGAINST GENDER-BASED HARASSMENT IN THE WORKPLACE. IN OTHER WORDS, IT BECAME ILLEGAL TO HARASS WOMEN JUST BECAUSE THEY WERE WOMEN.

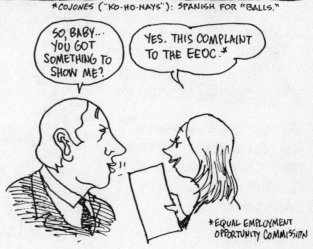

*EQUAL EMPLOYMENT OPPORTUNITY COMMISSION

GENDER-BASED HARASSMENT NEEDN'T BE SEXUAL. THERE ARE PLENTY OF WAYS TO ANNOY OR INTIMIDATE SOMEONE, BUT THE HEADLINE-GRABBERS, NATURALLY, ARE THE CASES INVOLVING SEX: PERSISTENT COME-ONS, LEWD JOKES, SEXUAL REMARKS, ETC...

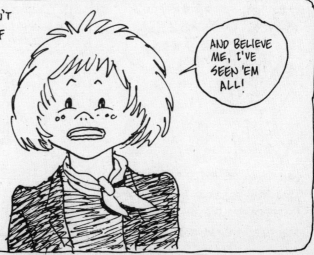

207

These jokes and comments may look different to the two sexes. A man may think he's only being playful and can't understand why a woman takes offense.

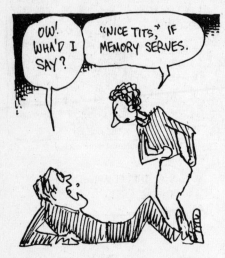

At least, that's what he may say... but in reality, somewhere deep inside, his feelings may be vengeful, hostile, and misogynistic!

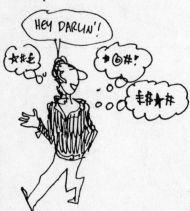

(And also, as noted in Chapter 6, men may mistake a woman's friendliness for sexual interest and encouragement.)

Women, meanwhile, may see a man's flirtatious compliment as merely one more in a long line of sexual intrusions she has to endure every day.

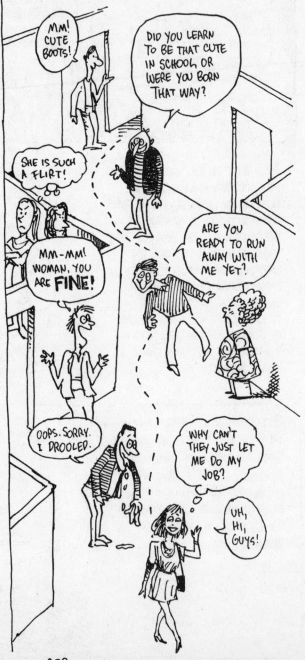

WHERE DOES ACCEPTABLE FLIRTING LEAVE OFF AND SEXUAL HARASSMENT BEGIN? THESE QUESTIONS MUST BE ANSWERED:

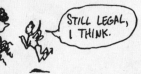 DO THE TWO PEOPLE HAVE EQUAL POWER? IF A BOSS OR PROFESSOR ASKS A SUBORDINATE OR STUDENT FOR SEXUAL FAVORS — OR EVEN A DATE — WHAT ARE THE POSSIBLE CONSEQUENCE?

WHAT ABOUT THE WOMAN WHO FLIRTS WITH HER BOSS?

STILL LEGAL, I THINK.

 WAS THE REMARK OR APPROACH REASONABLE AND POLITE, OR WERE THERE INAPPROPRIATE LANGUAGE, GESTURES, TOUCHING, ETC.?

DOES THE BEHAVIOR PERSIST, EVEN IF IT'S CLEARLY UNWELCOME?

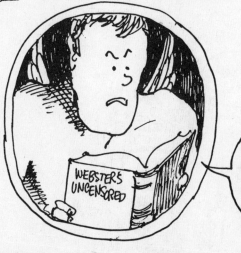

WEBSTER'S UNCENSORED

REMEMBER, POTENTIAL HARASSERS, "NO" MEANS **NO!!**

IF THE PERSON REALLY MEANS "MAYBE," BACK OFF ANYWAY! MAYBE SHE (OR HE) WILL LEARN TO BE MORE DIRECT IN THE FUTURE. ANYWAY, IT'S NOT YOUR JOB TO INTERPRET THE MEANING OF "NO." TAKE IT AT FACE VALUE.

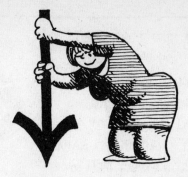

NOW THAT WOMEN HAVE MOVED INTO POSITIONS OF AUTHORITY, THEY TOO ARE IN A POSITION TO SEXUALLY HARASS THEIR MALE SUBORDINATES. THERE CAN ALSO BE SAME-SEX SEXUAL HARASSMENT.

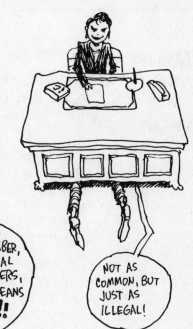

NOT AS COMMON, BUT JUST AS ILLEGAL!

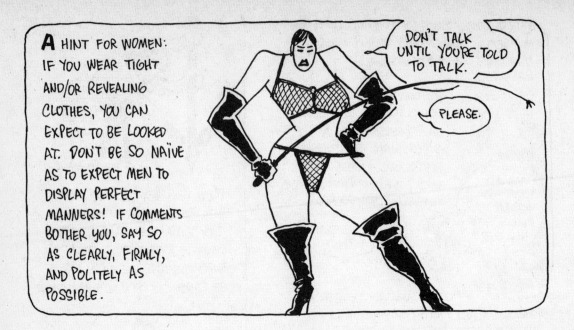

A HINT FOR WOMEN: IF YOU WEAR TIGHT AND/OR REVEALING CLOTHES, YOU CAN EXPECT TO BE LOOKED AT. DON'T BE SO NAÏVE AS TO EXPECT MEN TO DISPLAY PERFECT MANNERS! IF COMMENTS BOTHER YOU, SAY SO AS CLEARLY, FIRMLY, AND POLITELY AS POSSIBLE.

MEN: TRY TO RESPECT THE FACT THAT WOMEN OFTEN GET MORE SEXUAL ATTENTION THAN THEY WANT. AND REMEMBER, IT IS NEVER ALL RIGHT FOR A MAN TO TOUCH A WOMAN WITHOUT HER CONSENT, EVEN IF SHE'S AS NAKED AS LADY GODIVA!!

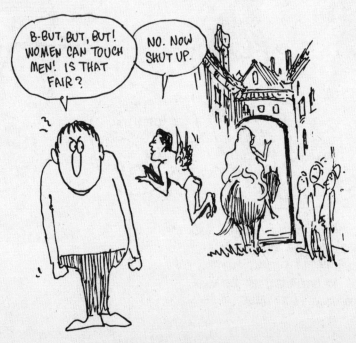

210

THE PUNISHMENT FOR SEXUAL HARASSMENT IS RARELY PRISON. RATHER THE LAW HOLDS COMPANIES AND COLLEGES RESPONSIBLE FOR INFRACTIONS THAT OCCUR UNDER THEIR AUSPICES. FINES MAY BE LEVIED, CLASS-ACTION LAWSUITS FILED, AND GENDER-SENSITIVITY WORKSHOPS ORDERED BY A COURT.

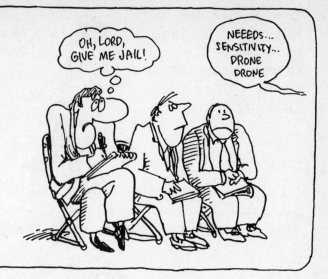

THE IDEA IS TO TEACH MEN TO BE SENSITIVE TO WOMEN'S POINT OF VIEW...

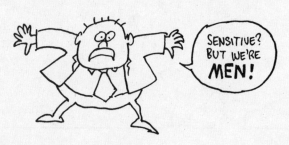

AND HELP MEN DEVELOP SOME NON-SEXUAL WAYS TO INTERACT WITH WOMEN.

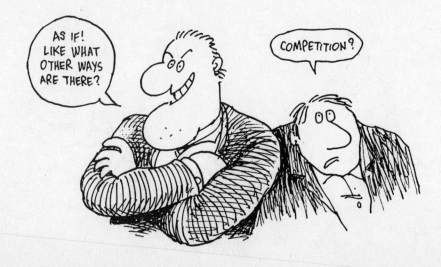

TO PROTECT THEMSELVES, MANY COMPANIES AND COLLEGES ARE QUICK TO DISCIPLINE EMPLOYEES OR STUDENTS WHO ARE ACCUSED OF SEXUAL HARASSMENT.

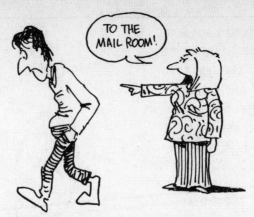

IT REALLY DOES PAY TO BE SENSITIVE TO THE ISSUE.

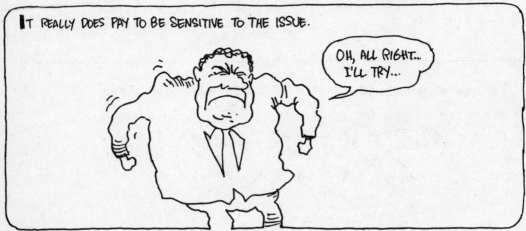

AND WHO KNOWS? MAYBE A DOSE OF GOOD MANNERS — WHAT ELSE DOES ANYONE WANT, AFTER ALL? — WILL MAKE EVERYONE A LITTLE HAPPIER AND MORE RELAXED!

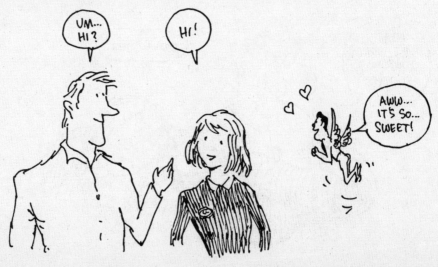

·CHAPTER 12·
PROBLEMS AND SOLUTIONS

During sex, a lot of stuff can come up... or maybe not...

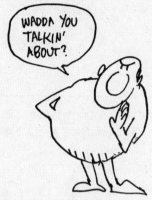

Most of us experience sexual difficulties at one time or another.

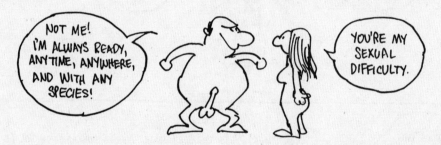

We may not be interested when our partner is, or vice versa, our attention may wander when it isn't supposed to, or our body just doesn't want to cooperate, for some reason.

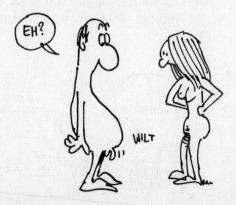

Sometimes these problems pass quickly, maybe after a good night's sleep, but sometimes they last longer and cause trouble. If so, there are two basic options: ignore the problem and hope it goes away, or talk it over with your partner.

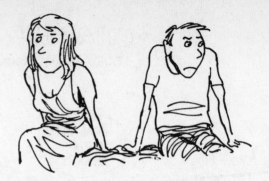

When the conversation is too difficult, or it doesn't seem to be enough, it may help to turn to a counselor, a physician, or a sex therapist like our old friend, **MERRY BUXOME.**

HI THERE! WANT TO GET "FIXED"?

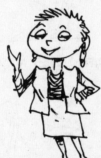

ONLY KIDDING, HEH HEH...

WHAT IN THE NAME OF THE SACRED GROVE OF GUM TREES IS A **SEX THERA-PIST?**

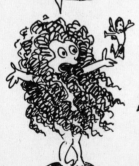

Sex therapists usually have a background in social work, psychology, or counseling, with extra training in human sexuality. We'll talk more about them a little later in the chapter. Meanwhile, Merry can guide us through some of the mental and physical problems she's encountered in her practice.

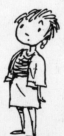

I'M ONLY TRYING TO HELP!

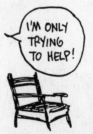

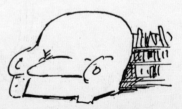

THERAPISTS TEND TO DISTINGUISH BETWEEN PHYSICAL PROBLEMS, OR **DYSFUNCTIONS**, AND PSYCHOLOGICAL PROBLEMS, OR **DISORDERS**.

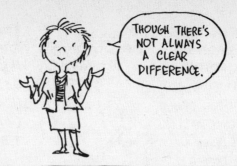

A COMMON DISORDER FOR BOTH MEN AND WOMEN IS **HSD**, OR HYPOACTIVE SEXUAL DESIRE — A SCIENTIFIC NAME FOR LOSING ALL INTEREST IN SEX.

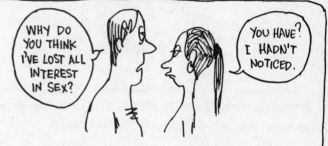

AS WE NOTED IN CHAPTER 5, MALE TESTOSTERONE LEVELS ARE HIGH EARLY IN A RELATIONSHIP, WHEN THERE'S STILL A SENSE OF CHALLENGE. LATER, TESTOSTERONE LEVELS DROP... MEN FEEL LESS SEXY... AND SO THEY'RE LESS OF A TURN-ON TO THEIR PARTNERS TOO...

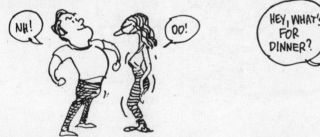

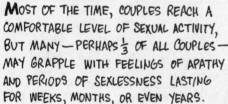

MOST OF THE TIME, COUPLES REACH A COMFORTABLE LEVEL OF SEXUAL ACTIVITY, BUT MANY — PERHAPS $\frac{1}{3}$ OF ALL COUPLES — MAY GRAPPLE WITH FEELINGS OF APATHY AND PERIODS OF SEXLESSNESS LASTING FOR WEEKS, MONTHS, OR EVEN YEARS.

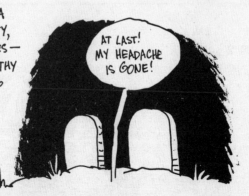

SOMETIMES HSD HAS A PHYSICAL CAUSE. EXTREME FATIGUE, SOME PRESCRIPTION DRUGS, AND HEAVY DRINKING CAN ALL DEPRESS SEXUAL DESIRE.

IT CAN ALSO STEM FROM DEEP ANXIETY ABOUT SEX OR HOSTILITY (ACKNOWLEDGED OR NOT) TOWARD THE PARTNER.

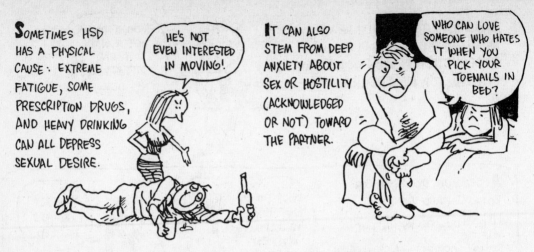

IF PHYSICAL CAUSES CAN BE RULED OUT, A PERSON WITH PERSISTENT HSD WILL NEED TO LOOK INWARD FOR REASONS. THIS IS WHERE A SEX THERAPIST MAY BE ABLE TO HELP.

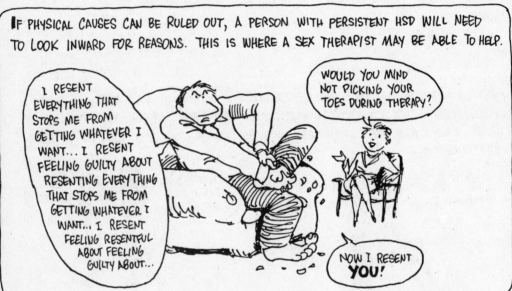

HAVING KIDS CAN DEPRESS SEXUAL DESIRE AS WELL.

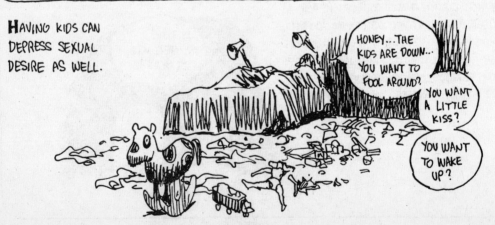

MORE SEVERE THAN MERE LOSS OF
INTEREST IS

SEXUAL AVERSION.

IN THIS DISORDER, THE SUFFERER
FEARS SEX SO MUCH THAT EVEN A
SIMPLE TOUCH OR KISS CAN BRING
ON SWEATING, NAUSEA, OR VOMITING.

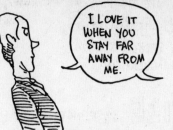
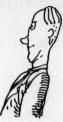

I LOVE IT WHEN YOU STAY FAR AWAY FROM ME.

SEXUAL AVERSION CAN BE THE RESULT OF CHILDHOOD TRAUMA, SUCH AS SEXUAL ABUSE OR
PARENTAL HOSTILITY, OR EXTREME BODY-IMAGE PROBLEMS (OBESITY, ACNE, ETC.). HOW MUCH
A THERAPIST CAN HELP DEPENDS ON THE SEVERITY OF THE CONDITION, THE THERAPIST'S
SKILL, AND (POSSIBLY MOST IMPORTANT) THE PERSON'S WILLINGNESS TO WORK ON THE
PROBLEM.

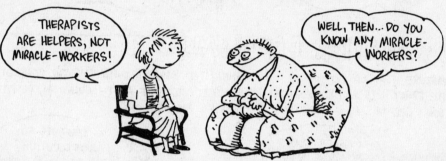

THERAPISTS ARE HELPERS, NOT MIRACLE-WORKERS!

WELL, THEN... DO YOU KNOW ANY MIRACLE-WORKERS?

GAYS AND LESBIANS
WHO EXPERIENCE THESE
"DESIRE DISORDERS" MAY
BE STRUGGLING WITH
INTERNALIZED HOMOPHOBIA.
UNABLE FULLY TO SHAKE
OFF SOCIETY'S NEGATIVE
JUDGMENTS, AMBIVALENT
ABOUT THEIR SEXUAL
ORIENTATION, THEY MAY
FEEL PARALYZED WHEN
IT COMES TO SEXUAL
EXPRESSION.

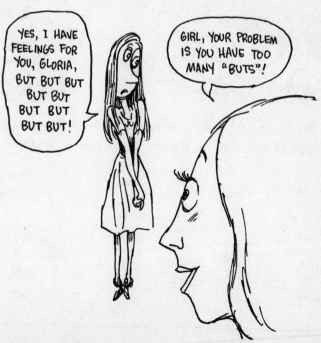

YES, I HAVE FEELINGS FOR YOU, GLORIA, BUT BUT BUT BUT BUT BUT BUT BUT BUT!

GIRL, YOUR PROBLEM IS YOU HAVE TOO MANY "BUTS"!

AND THEN THERE ARE THE PHYSICAL PROBLEMS, OR

DYSFUNCTIONS.

THESE INCLUDE PROBLEMS WITH ERECTION AND EJACULATION.

ANNOY YOUR FRIENDS! CHALLENGE THEM TO NAME A WORD CONTAINING THE LETTERS "YSF!"

ERECTILE DYSFUNCTION — IT USED TO BE CALLED **IMPOTENCE** — IS AN INABILITY TO GET OR SUSTAIN AN ERECTION. THIS CAN BE CRUSHING TO THE FRAGILE MALE EGO!

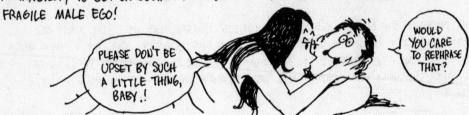

PLEASE DON'T BE UPSET BY SUCH A LITTLE THING, BABY.!

WOULD YOU CARE TO REPHRASE THAT?

EJACULATION PROBLEMS

PREMATURE EJACULATION — "COMING EARLY." (SOME INCONSIDERATE MEN DON'T SEE THIS AS A PROBLEM.)

INHIBITED EJACULATION MEANS THE COMPLETE INABILITY TO HAVE AN EJACULATION, DESPITE HAVING AN ERECTION.

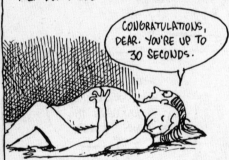

CONGRATULATIONS, DEAR. YOU'RE UP TO 30 SECONDS.

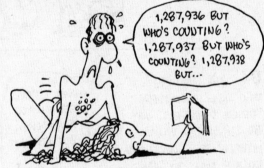

1,287,936 BUT WHO'S COUNTING? 1,287,937 BUT WHO'S COUNTING? 1,287,938 BUT...

DELAYED EJACULATION IS WHEN THE MAN CAN REACH ORGASM ONLY AFTER PROLONGED STIMULATION, LIKE 40 MINUTES OF CONTINUOUS THRUSTING OR STROKING.

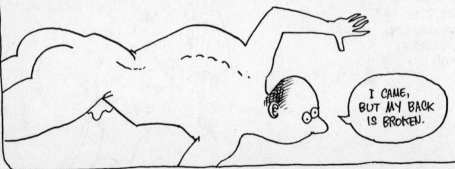

I CAME, BUT MY BACK IS BROKEN.

SOME FEMALE SEXUAL DYSFUNCTIONS:

ANORGASMIA

IS THE INABILITY TO REACH ORGASM.

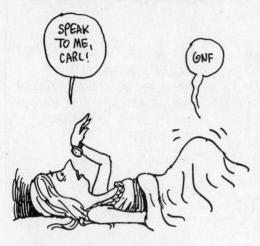

VAGINISMUS

IS AN INVOLUNTARY SPASM OF THE VAGINAL MUSCLES, PREVENTING PENETRATION.

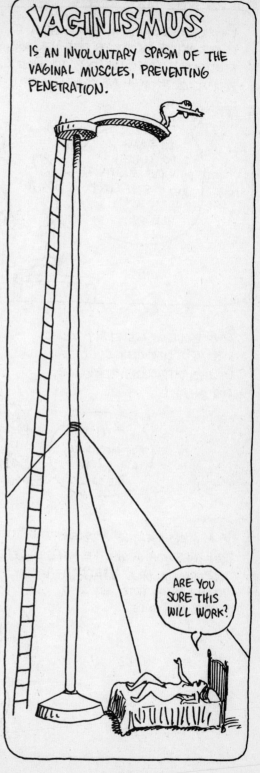

DISPAREUNIA

IS PAIN DURING INTERCOURSE.

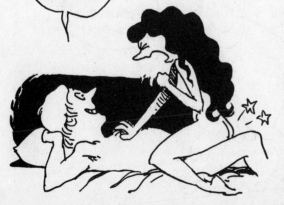

PHYSICAL PROBLEMS CAN HAVE PHYSICAL OR PSYCHOLOGICAL CAUSES. POSSIBLE PHYSICAL CAUSES INCLUDE ALCOHOL OR DRUG USE, SOME CHRONIC DISEASES LIKE DIABETES, AND HORMONE FLUCTUATIONS (IN EITHER SEX). THE FIRST STEP IN TREATING A SEXUAL DYSFUNCTION IS A MEDICAL CHECK-UP — AND BE SURE TO TELL THE DOCTOR EVERYTHING, NO MATTER HOW EMBARRASSING.

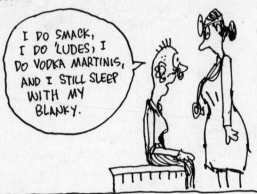

I DO SMACK, I DO 'LUDES, I DO VODKA MARTINIS, AND I STILL SLEEP WITH MY BLANKY.

FOR WOMEN, THE CHECK-UP SHOULD INCLUDE A PELVIC EXAM FOR ENDOMETRIOSIS, UTERINE CYSTS OR TUMORS, CLITORAL ADHESIONS, AN OBSTRUCTED HYMEN, OR SCAR TISSUE.

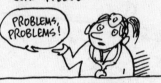

PROBLEMS, PROBLEMS!

SOME PROBLEMS ARE EASILY SOLVED: A SIMPLE LUBRICANT CAN OFTEN RELIEVE DIFFICULT INTERCOURSE, FOR EXAMPLE.

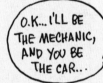

O.K... I'LL BE THE MECHANIC, AND YOU BE THE CAR...

IF A MAN'S ERECTILE PROBLEMS ARE DUE TO ILLNESS OR INJURY, HE MAY CONSIDER THE "ERECTION DRUG" **VIAGRA.** IF THAT DOESN'T WORK, THERE ARE ALSO PENILE IMPLANTS.

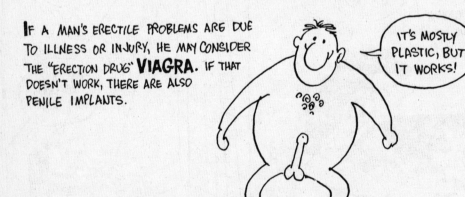

IT'S MOSTLY PLASTIC, BUT IT WORKS!

220

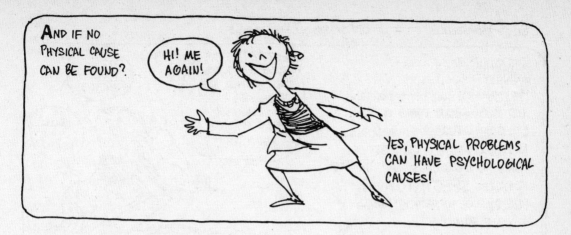

AND IF NO PHYSICAL CAUSE CAN BE FOUND?

HI! ME AGAIN!

YES, PHYSICAL PROBLEMS CAN HAVE PSYCHOLOGICAL CAUSES!

FOR EXAMPLE, SOME PEOPLE ARE JUST TOO STRESSED OUT TO PERFORM SEXUALLY.

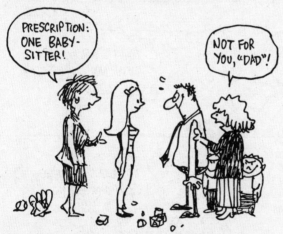

PRESCRIPTION: ONE BABY-SITTER!

NOT FOR YOU, "DAD"!

MANY WOMEN'S ANORGASMIA MAY BE DUE TO SIMPLE IGNORANCE. HER PARTNER MAY NOT KNOW HOW TO STIMULATE HER CLITORIS, AND THE WOMAN MAY BE TOO SQUEAMISH OR INEXPERIENCED TO SHOW HIM WHAT TO DO.

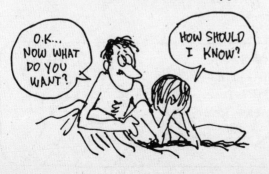

O.K... NOW WHAT DO YOU WANT?

HOW SHOULD I KNOW?

THEN THERE'S "SITUATIONAL ANORGASMIA." SOME WOMEN CAN HAVE ORGASMS ONLY IN CERTAIN SITUATIONS (WHILE MASTURBATING, FOR EXAMPLE) BUT NEVER IN OTHERS.

OO-OU-OO-OO-OO OO-AH-AH-AH!

HOW LONG HAS IT BEEN SINCE YOU COULD ONLY ACHIEVE ORGASM HERE IN THE OFFICE?

ANXIETY:

PERFORMANCE ANXIETY — WORRYING TOO MUCH ABOUT DOING IT "RIGHT" — CAN STOP A PERSON FROM DOING ANYTHING AT ALL. THE HABIT OF "LOOKING OVER ONE'S OWN SHOULDER" IS CALLED **SPECTATORING.** PERFORMANCE ANXIETY IS MOSTLY A MALE PROBLEM.

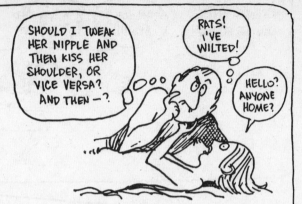

SOME ANXIETY CAN BE BASED ON A GENEROUS DESIRE TO PLEASE OUR PARTNER, BUT WHEN DESIRE TO PLEASE BECOMES FEAR OF DISPLEASING — THAT'S WHEN TROUBLE CAN START!

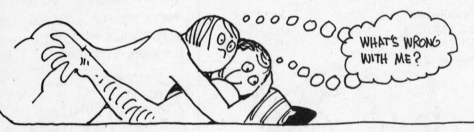

INNER CONFLICTS

OF VARIOUS KINDS CAN LEAD TO EVERYTHING FROM ERECTILE PROBLEMS TO VAGINISMUS AND ANORGASMIA. OUR GNAWING DOUBTS AND UNRESOLVED CONFLICTS CAN COME FROM MANY SOURCES. FOR EXAMPLE, A RIGID, PRUDISH UPBRINGING MAY HAVE LEFT US WITH LINGERING FEELINGS THAT PHYSICAL PLEASURE IS TABOO...

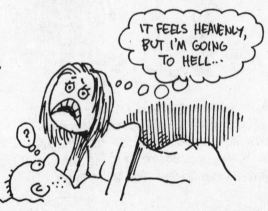

OR WE MAY NOT BE OVER AN EX (OR SEVERAL EXES!).

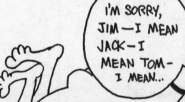

THE PSYCHOLOGICAL AFTERMATH OF **SEXUAL ASSAULT** CAN LEAD TO DYSFUNCTION AS WELL. PEOPLE WHO EXPERIENCE REPEATED SEXUAL ABUSE AS CHILDREN ARE MORE LIKELY TO AVOID SEX, LACK DESIRE, AND HAVE PROBLEMS REACHING ORGASM.

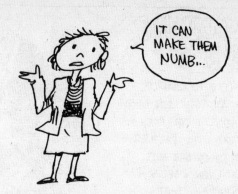

IT CAN MAKE THEM NUMB...

PSYCHOTHERAPISTS CLAIM SOME SUCCESS IN HELPING COUPLES IN WHICH ONE PARTNER SUFFERED ABUSE AS A CHILD. THE THERAPIST'S ROLE IS TO HELP BOTH PARTNERS UNDERSTAND THE ROLE PLAYED BY THE ABUSE IN THE DYNAMICS OF THE CURRENT RELATIONSHIP.

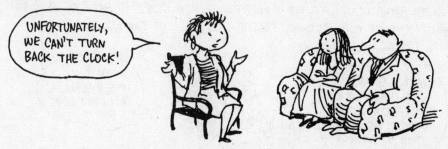

UNFORTUNATELY, WE CAN'T TURN BACK THE CLOCK!

ADULT RAPE VICTIMS MAY ALSO HAVE PROBLEMS, AS THEY MAY COME TO ASSOCIATE ALL SEXUAL RELATIONS WITH THEIR ONE HORRIBLE EXPERIENCE. A RAPE VICTIM USUALLY TAKES SOME TIME TO GET OVER IT, AND IT HELPS IF HER PARTNER IS SYMPATHETIC AND PATIENT.

O.K., SWEETHEART... WHENEVER YOU'RE READY...

PEPPER SPRAY

223

RELATIONSHIP PROBLEMS

CAN ALSO LEAD TO TROUBLES THAT LOOK AN AWFUL LOT LIKE DYSFUNCTIONS. MAYBE SOMETHING ABOUT THE PARTNER— THE WAY HE OR SHE ACTS, LOOKS, OR EVEN SMELLS— MAY BE STOPPING THAT ORGASM OR MAKING THAT ERECTION DROOP.

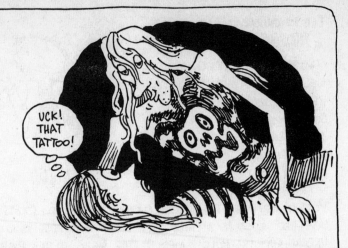

UCK! THAT TATTOO!

SOMETIMES WE MAY NOT EVEN BE AWARE OF WHAT THE PROBLEM IS... OR WE MAY BE UNWILLING TO BRING IT UP...OR WE MAY THINK TALKING WON'T DO ANY GOOD... OR WE DON'T WANT TO HURT OUR PARTNER'S FEELINGS... OR ALL OF THE ABOVE.

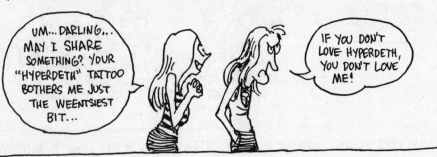

UM...DARLING... MAY I SHARE SOMETHING? YOUR "HYPERDETH" TATTOO BOTHERS ME JUST THE WEENTSIEST BIT...

IF YOU DON'T LOVE HYPERDETH, YOU DON'T LOVE ME!

IF THE DISCUSSION SEEMS TOO HARD, COUPLES THERAPY MAY HELP. THE THERAPIST WILL PROBABLY POINT OUT THAT PROBLEMS LIKE THESE HAVE TWO SIDES, AND SHE WILL TRY TO FIND A MIDDLE GROUND.

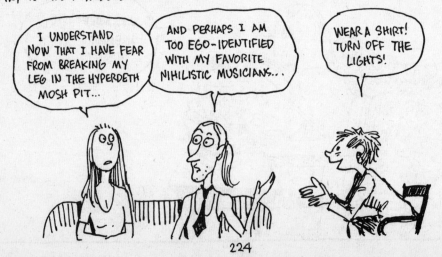

I UNDERSTAND NOW THAT I HAVE FEAR FROM BREAKING MY LEG IN THE HYPERDETH MOSH PIT...

AND PERHAPS I AM TOO EGO-IDENTIFIED WITH MY FAVORITE NIHILISTIC MUSICIANS...

WEAR A SHIRT! TURN OFF THE LIGHTS!

MORE ABOUT **THERAPY** 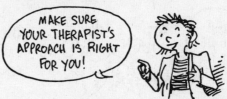 YAK YAK YAK

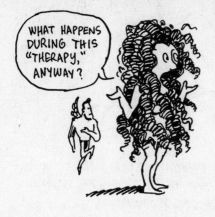

WHAT HAPPENS DURING THIS "THERAPY," ANYWAY?

SINCE THERAPISTS HAVE DIFFERENT BACKGROUNDS, THEY MAY NOT ALL APPROACH PROBLEMS THE SAME WAY. "COGNITIVE-BEHAVIORAL" THERAPISTS FOCUS ON CHANGING WHAT WE DO AND HOW WE THINK ABOUT OUR SEX LIVES. THOSE WITH A MORE "PSYCHOSEXUAL" APPROACH WANT TO DELVE DEEPER INTO THE ROOTS OF OUR INNER LIVES.

MAKE SURE YOUR THERAPIST'S APPROACH IS RIGHT FOR YOU!

AND DON'T WORRY TOO MUCH! THERAPY IS MOSTLY TALK. CHANCES ARE, EVERYONE KEEPS THEIR CLOTHES ON, AND NOBODY GETS HORIZONTAL.

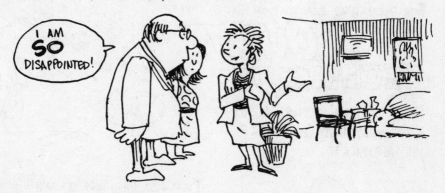

I AM **SO** DISAPPOINTED!

SOMETIMES TALK IS ALL IT TAKES: AIRING THE ISSUES, EXPOSING BURIED RESENTMENTS, AND EXPLORING RELATIONSHIP DYNAMICS MAY BE ENOUGH TO GIVE PEOPLE THE MEANS TO REMEDY THEIR SITUATION. OR MAYBE NOT!

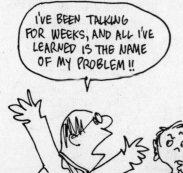

I'VE BEEN TALKING FOR WEEKS, AND ALL I'VE LEARNED IS THE NAME OF MY PROBLEM!!

IF TALK ISN'T ENOUGH, THE THERAPIST MAY GIVE SPECIFIC PHYSICAL "HOMEWORK ASSIGNMENTS," LIKE THE ONES DESIGNED BY THE PIONEERING SEX THERAPISTS WILLIAM **MASTERS** AND VIRGINIA **JOHNSON.**

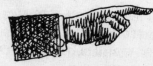

225

SENSATE FOCUS

IS THE SAME THING WE DESCRIBED IN CHAPTER 8: GIVING AND RECEIVING PLEASURE THROUGH TOUCH WITHOUT STRIVING FOR ORGASM. BESIDES TEACHING EACH OTHER WHAT'S AROUSING, SENSATE FOCUS ALSO HELPS PARTNERS GET COMFORTABLE AND RELAXED ABOUT TOUCHING EACH OTHER.

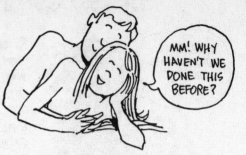

MM! WHY HAVEN'T WE DONE THIS BEFORE?

OBOY! NOW WE GET TO TOUCH IT!

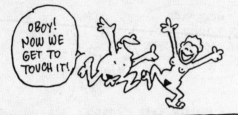

ONCE EVERYONE IS COMFORTABLE, THEY CAN MOVE ON TO TECHNIQUES DESIGNED FOR SPECIFIC PROBLEMS.

FOR PREMATURE EJACULATION, FOR EXAMPLE, THERE'S THE "SQUEEZE" TECHNIQUE.

FIRST, THE MAN IS BROUGHT TO ERECTION BY HAND (HIS OWN OR HIS PARTNER'S).

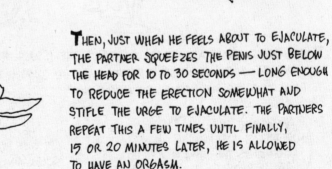

OO!

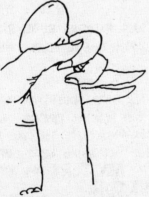

THEN, JUST WHEN HE FEELS ABOUT TO EJACULATE, THE PARTNER SQUEEZES THE PENIS JUST BELOW THE HEAD FOR 10 TO 30 SECONDS — LONG ENOUGH TO REDUCE THE ERECTION SOMEWHAT AND STIFLE THE URGE TO EJACULATE. THE PARTNERS REPEAT THIS A FEW TIMES UNTIL FINALLY, 15 OR 20 MINUTES LATER, HE IS ALLOWED TO HAVE AN ORGASM.

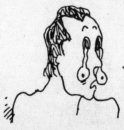

NEXT TIME, SWEETIE, TRY NOT TO SQUEEZE QUITE SO HARD!

AFTER SEVERAL DAYS' PRACTICE, THE COUPLE MOVES ON TO INTERCOURSE WITH THE WOMAN ON TOP SO SHE CAN CONTROL THE PACE.

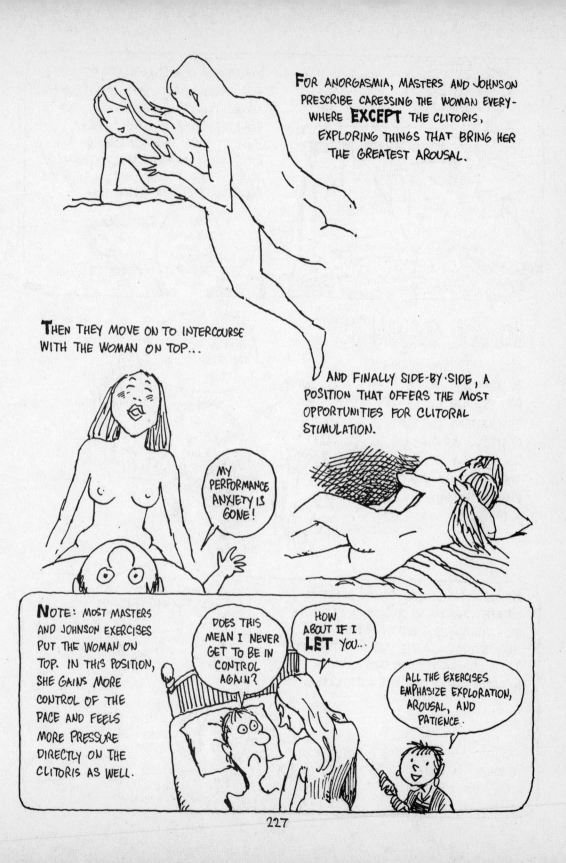

FOR ANORGASMIA, MASTERS AND JOHNSON PRESCRIBE CARESSING THE WOMAN EVERY- WHERE **EXCEPT** THE CLITORIS, EXPLORING THINGS THAT BRING HER THE GREATEST AROUSAL.

THEN THEY MOVE ON TO INTERCOURSE WITH THE WOMAN ON TOP...

AND FINALLY SIDE-BY-SIDE, A POSITION THAT OFFERS THE MOST OPPORTUNITIES FOR CLITORAL STIMULATION.

MY PERFORMANCE ANXIETY IS GONE!

NOTE: MOST MASTERS AND JOHNSON EXERCISES PUT THE WOMAN ON TOP. IN THIS POSITION, SHE GAINS MORE CONTROL OF THE PACE AND FEELS MORE PRESSURE DIRECTLY ON THE CLITORIS AS WELL.

DOES THIS MEAN I NEVER GET TO BE IN CONTROL AGAIN?

HOW ABOUT IF I **LET** YOU...

ALL THE EXERCISES EMPHASIZE EXPLORATION, AROUSAL, AND PATIENCE.

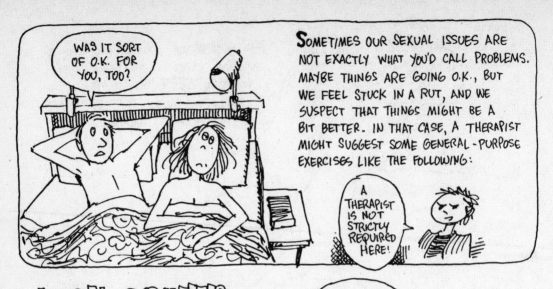

SOMETIMES OUR SEXUAL ISSUES ARE NOT EXACTLY WHAT YOU'D CALL PROBLEMS. MAYBE THINGS ARE GOING O.K., BUT WE FEEL STUCK IN A RUT, AND WE SUSPECT THAT THINGS MIGHT BE A BIT BETTER. IN THAT CASE, A THERAPIST MIGHT SUGGEST SOME GENERAL-PURPOSE EXERCISES LIKE THE FOLLOWING:

Was it sort of O.K. for you, too?

A THERAPIST IS NOT STRICTLY REQUIRED HERE!

KEGEL SQUEEZES

ARE A MUSCULAR EXERCISE. TO DO KEGELS, SIMPLY TIGHTEN AND RELEASE THE MUSCLES THAT CONTROL THE FLOW OF URINE. YOU CAN DO KEGELS FAST OR SLOW, TEN AT A TIME, FOR FIVE OR TEN SESSIONS A DAY.

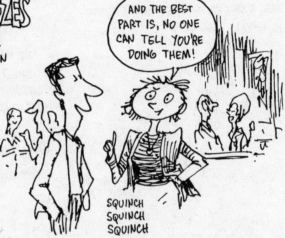

AND THE BEST PART IS, NO ONE CAN TELL YOU'RE DOING THEM!

SQUINCH
SQUINCH
SQUINCH

KEGELS OFFER SEVERAL SEXUAL BENEFITS: GREATER AWARENESS OF SENSATIONS IN THE AREA, INCREASED BLOOD CIRCULATION AND HEIGHTENED SENSATION DURING INTERCOURSE AS THE VAGINA IS TIGHTENED. (THOSE SQUEEZES CAN UP THE PARTNER'S AROUSAL TOO!)

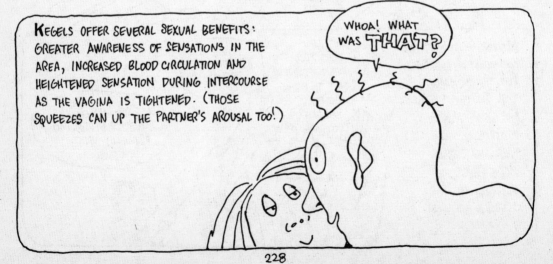

WHOA! WHAT WAS THAT?

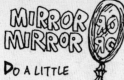

MIRROR MIRROR

Do a little uncritical self-examination. Use a full-length mirror and a hand-held mirror for a view of everything! The idea here is to become more aware of and comfortable with your own body.

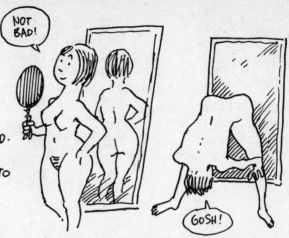

NOT BAD!

GOSH!

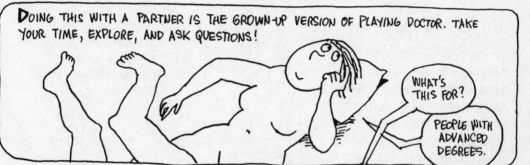

Doing this with a partner is the grown-up version of playing doctor. Take your time, explore, and ask questions!

WHAT'S THIS FOR?

PEOPLE WITH ADVANCED DEGREES.

WATER PLAY

If it's good enough for fish, why not for people? Try it in a bath or shower.

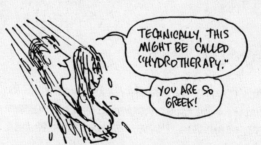

TECHNICALLY, THIS MIGHT BE CALLED "HYDROTHERAPY."

YOU ARE SO GREEK!

GREASE

Massage with oils, lotions, or lubricants, with or without orgasm as a goal. (But remember that oil makes latex condoms disintegrate.)

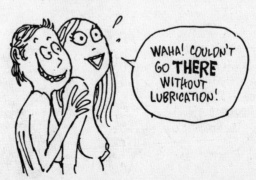

WAHA! COULDN'T GO **THERE** WITHOUT LUBRICATION!

VISUAL AIDS:

ALONE OR IN PAIRS,
CONSIDER EROTICA, IN
PRINT OR ON VIDEO.
LET YOUR PARTNER KNOW
WHAT TURNS YOU ON.
(TRY TO KEEP IT LEGAL.)

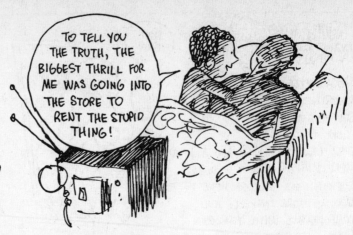

SECRETS:

IF THE LEVEL OF TRUST
BETWEEN YOU IS HIGH, SHARE
YOUR SECRET FANTASIES. YOU'LL
GROW CLOSER AS A RESULT
OF REVEALING SOMETHING SO
INTIMATE... AND WHO KNOWS?
MAYBE SOMEBODY'S DREAMS
MAY COME TRUE!

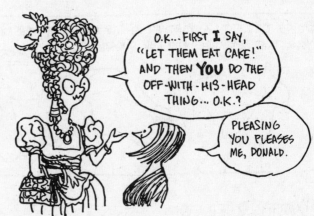

TOYS

LET'S FACE IT: IT'S AN INDUSTRY! AN AMAZING ARRAY OF "EROTIC AIDS" IS
COMMERCIALLY AVAILABLE: VIBRATORS, DILDOS, "COCK RINGS," NIPPLE CLIPS, FUR-LINED
HANDCUFFS, HARNESSES, PLUGS, CONDOMS WITH FRILLS... YOU NAME IT; SOMEBODY
SELLS IT!

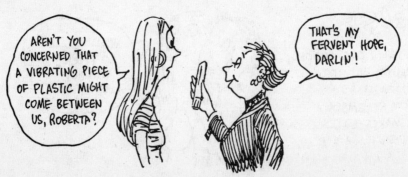

THE BIG QUESTION IN ALL THIS HAS TO BE: WHAT ARE WE TRYING TO ACCOMPLISH HERE? WHAT'S THE POINT? THE GOAL OF ALL THIS EXPLORATION?

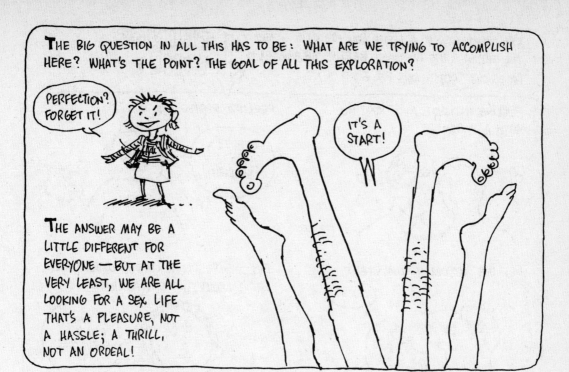

PERFECTION? FORGET IT!

IT'S A START!

THE ANSWER MAY BE A LITTLE DIFFERENT FOR EVERYONE — BUT AT THE VERY LEAST, WE ARE ALL LOOKING FOR A SEX LIFE THAT'S A PLEASURE, NOT A HASSLE; A THRILL, NOT AN ORDEAL!

WHAT ARE SOME BASIC INGREDIENTS OF A HOT AND TASTY SEX LIFE?

* ACCURATE INFORMATION ABOUT SEXUALITY, OUR OWN AND OUR PARTNER'S

* A VIEW OF SEX AS PLEASURE, NOT PERFORMANCE

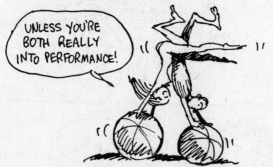

UNLESS YOU'RE BOTH REALLY INTO PERFORMANCE!

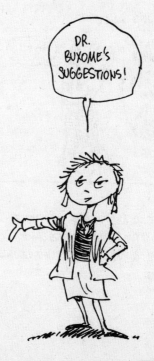

DR. BUXOME'S SUGGESTIONS!

* GOOD COMMUNICATION WITH OUR PARTNER ABOUT NEEDS AND FEELINGS.

* UNDERSTANDING, ACCEPTING, AND APPRECIATING THE DIFFERENCES AND SIMILARITIES BETWEEN OUR PARTNERS AND OURSELVES.

WE MIGHT ALSO DO A LITTLE SOUL-SEARCHING ABOUT THE THINGS THAT THERAPIST **BERNIE ZILBERGELD** CALLS OUR "CONDITIONS FOR GOOD SEX." **THINGS LIKE:**

FEELING INTIMATE AND TRUSTING WITH A PARTNER

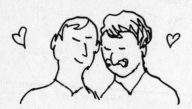

FEELING RESTED AND ALERT

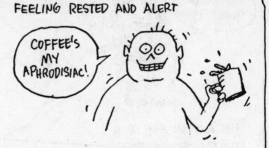

COFFEE'S MY APHRODISIAC!

FEELING SEXUALLY COMPETENT

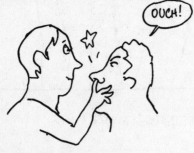

OUCH!

FEELING POSITIVE (SAFE, COMFORTABLE, ETC.) ABOUT THE ENVIRONMENT

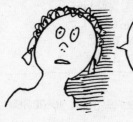

I LIKE CROWDED ELEVATORS! SO?

FEELING AROUSED

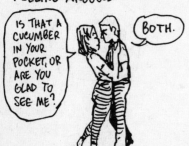

IS THAT A CUCUMBER IN YOUR POCKET, OR ARE YOU GLAD TO SEE ME?

BOTH.

FEELING THAT OUR PARTNER APPRECIATES US.

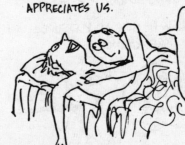

UM... IF IT'S NOT TOO MUCH TROUBLE, WOULD YOU MIND SAYING "WOW" AGAIN?

WE CAN ALL AGREE ON THOSE, BUT OTHER CONDITIONS ARE MORE A MATTER OF INDIVIDUAL TASTE.

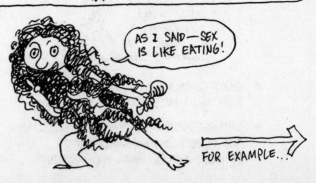

AS I SAID — SEX IS LIKE EATING!

FOR EXAMPLE...

232

HOT OR COLD?
LIGHTS ON OR LIGHTS OUT?
MORNING OR EVENING? MUSIC
OR SILENCE? NUDITY OR COSTUMES?
TENDER WORDS OR X-RATED BARKS?
A GLASS OF WINE? A CUP OF COFFEE?
A BAG OF CHIPS? SLOW OR FAST?
KINKY OR "VANILLA"? VARIETY
OR FAMILIARITY? ENDLESS
TALKING, OR.....?

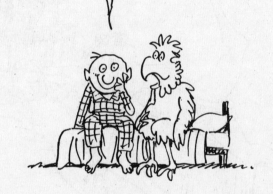

WE ALL HOPE
WE CAN FIND
SOMEONE WHOSE
CONDITIONS ARE
SIMILAR TO OUR
OWN.

WOOF! I CAN'T
BELIEVE YOU'RE A
SLOW-GOING, WINE-
DRINKING, VANILLA
MORNING BARKER
TOO!

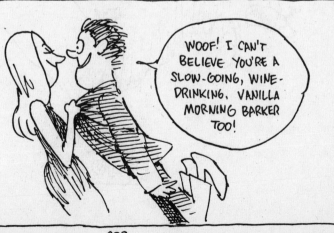

FROM THAT POINT ON, IT'S A FAIRLY SIMPLE MATTER
OF PATIENCE, OPENNESS, AND A CERTAIN WILLINGNESS
TO EXPLORE... OH, AND DON'T FORGET A SENSE
OF HUMOR!!

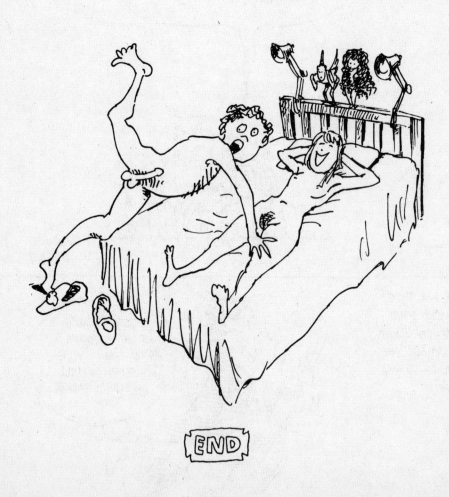

END

· BIBLIOGRAPHY ·

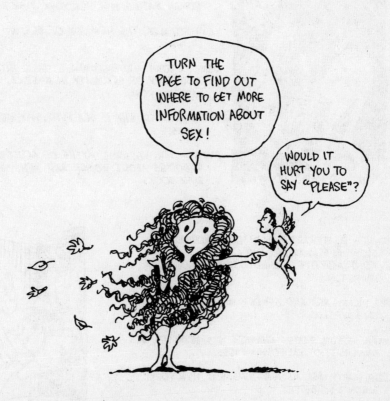

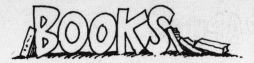# BOOKS

ACKERMAN, DIANE, *A NATURAL HISTORY OF LOVE*, 1994, NEW YORK, RANDOM HOUSE.

BARBACH, LONNIE, *FOR EACH OTHER: SHARING SEXUAL INTIMACY*, 1984, NEW YORK, BANTAM.

BLUM, DEBORAH, *SEX ON THE BRAIN*, 1997, NEW YORK, VIKING.

BOSTON WOMENS HEALTH BOOK COLLECTIVE, *OUR BODIES, OURSELVES: FOR THE NEW CENTURY*, 1998, NEW YORK, SIMON & SCHUSTER.

BULLOUGH, VERN L., AND BULLOUGH, BONNIE, *SEXUAL ATTITUDES THROUGHOUT THE AGES*, 1995, NEW YORK, PROMETHEUS BOOKS.

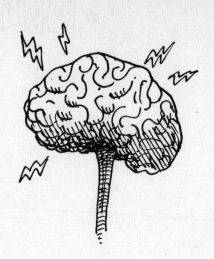

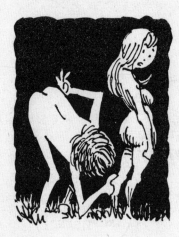

BUSS, DAVID M., *THE EVOLUTION OF DESIRE: STRATEGIES OF HUMAN MATING*, 1994, NEW YORK, BASIC BOOKS.

COMFORT, ALEX, *THE NEW JOY OF SEX*, 1991, NEW YORK, CROWN.

DEMILIO, JOHN, AND FREEDMAN, ESTELLE, *INTIMATE MATTERS: A HISTORY OF SEXUALITY IN AMERICA*, 1988, NEW YORK, HARPER & ROW.

DIAMOND, JARED, *WHY IS SEX FUN?*, 1997, NEW YORK, BASIC BOOKS.

FAUSTO-STERLING, ANNE, *MYTHS OF GENDER: BIOLOGICAL THEORIES ABOUT WOMEN AND MEN*, 1985, NEW YORK, BASIC BOOKS.

HATCHER, R., STEWART, F., TRUSSEL, J., KOWAL, D., GUEST, F., STEWART, G., AND CATES, W., *CONTRACEPTIVE TECHNOLOGY*, 1994, NEW YORK, IRVINGTON.

LIPS, HILARY, *SEX AND GENDER*, 1997, MOUNTAIN VIEW, CA, MAYFIELD.

LUKER, KRISTIN, *TAKING CHANCES*, 1975, BERKELEY, CA, UNIVERSITY OF CALIFORNIA PRESS.

KLEIN, MARTY, *ASK ME ANYTHING*, 1992, NEW YORK, SIMON & SCHUSTER.

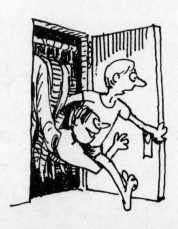

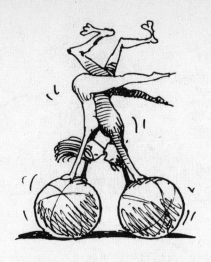

MICHAEL, ROBERT T., GAGNON, JOHN, LAUMANN, EDWARD, AND KOLATA, GINA, *SEX IN AMERICA: A DEFINITIVE SURVEY*, 1994, BOSTON, LITTLE, BROWN.

PECK, M. SCOTT, *THE ROAD LESS TRAVELED: A NEW PSYCHOLOGY OF LOVE, TRADITIONAL VALUES, AND SPIRITUAL GROWTH*, 1978, NEW YORK, SIMON & SCHUSTER.

PINKER, STEPHEN, *THE WAY THE MIND WORKS*, 1998, NEW YORK, NORTON.

SATIR, VIRGINIA, *THE NEW PEOPLEMAKING*, 1988, PALO ALTO, CA, SCIENCE AND BEHAVIOR BOOKS.

STERNBERG, ROBERT, AND BARNES, MICHAEL (EDS.), *THE PSYCHOLOGY OF LOVE*, 1988, NEW HAVEN, YALE UNIVERSITY PRESS.

STRONG, BRYAN, DEVAULT, CHRISTINE, AND SAYAD, BARBARA W., *HUMAN SEXUALITY: DIVERSITY IN CONTEMPORARY AMERICA, 3RD EDITION*, 1999, MOUNTAIN VIEW, CA, MAYFIELD.

SUGGS, DAVID, AND MIRACLE, ANDREW (EDS.), *CULTURE AND HUMAN SEXUALITY*, 1993, PACIFIC GROVE, CA, BROOKS/COLE.

SYMONS, DONALD, *THE EVOLUTION OF HUMAN SEXUALITY*, 1979, NEW YORK, OXFORD UNIVERSITY PRESS.

TANNAHILL, REAY, *SEX IN HISTORY*, REVISED EDITION, 1992, SCARBOROUGH HOUSE.

TANNEN, DEBORAH, *YOU JUST DONT UNDERSTAND: MEN AND WOMEN IN CONVERSATION*, 1990, NEW YORK, BALLANTINE.

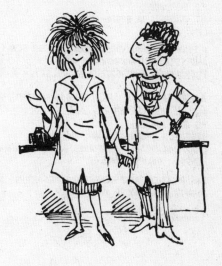

TISDALE, SALLIE, *TALK DIRTY TO ME: AN INTIMATE PHILOSOPHY OF SEX*, 1994, NEW YORK, FREE PRESS.

WEINBERG, MARTIN, WILLIAMS, COLIN, AND PRYOR, DOUGLAS, *DUAL ATTRACTION: UNDERSTANDING BISEXUALITY*, 1994, NEW YORK, OXFORD UNIVERSITY PRESS.

ZILBERGELD, BERNIE, *THE NEW MALE SEXUALITY*, 1992, NEW YORK, BANTAM BOOKS.

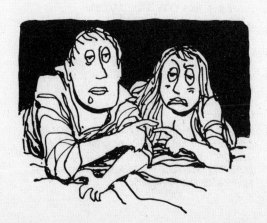

SOME JOURNALS ABOUT SEXUALITY:

AMERICAN JOURNAL OF PUBLIC HEALTH, ARCHIVES OF SEXUAL BEHAVIOR, FAMILY PLANNING PERSPECTIVES, JOURNAL OF HOMOSEXUALITY, JOURNAL OF SEX AND MARITAL THERAPY, JOURNAL OF SEX RESEARCH, SEX ROLES: A JOURNAL OF RESEARCH, SEXUALITIES, SIECUS REPORTS, AND WOMEN AND HEALTH.

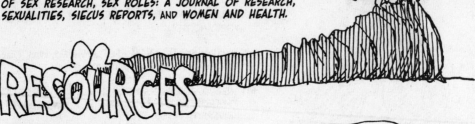

RESOURCES

AMERICAN ASSOCIATION OF SEX EDUCATORS, COUNSELORS AND THERAPISTS (AASECT)
P.O. BOX 238
MT. VERNON, IA 52314-0238
(319) 895-8407

A PROFESSIONAL ORGANIZATION FOR SEX THERAPISTS AND EDUCATORS. PROVIDES REFERRALS TO CERTIFIED THERAPISTS. PUBLISHES A NEWSLETTER AND JOURNAL.

AMERICAN SOCIAL HEALTH ASSOCIATION (ASHA) AND HERPES RESOURCE CENTER
P.O. BOX 13827
RESEARCH TRIANGLE PARK, NC 27709
(800) 653-HEALTH (653-4325), (919) 361-8400
HERPES: (919) 361-8488

INFORMATION AND REFERRALS REGARDING STDS. CONFIDENTIALITY IS MAINTAINED.

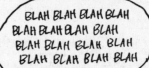

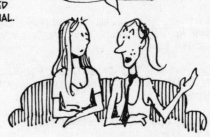

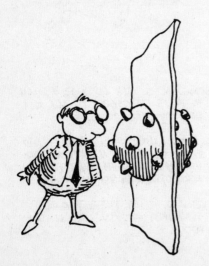

CDC NATIONAL HIV AND AIDS HOTLINE
(800) 342-AIDS (342-2437)
(800) 243-7889 (TTY, DEAF ACCESS)

INFORMATION AND REFERRALS FROM THE CENTER FOR DISEASE CONTROL AND PREVENTION.

NATIONAL ORGANIZATION OF CIRCUMCISION INFORMATION RESOURCE CENTERS (NOCIRC)
P.O. BOX 2512
SAN ANSELMO, CA 94979
(415) 488-9883

PROVIDES MEDICAL AND LEGAL INFORMATION ON CIRCUMCISION AND FEMALE GENITAL MUTILATION (OPPOSES ROUTINE HOSPITAL CIRCUMCISION). PAMPHLETS, NEWSLETTERS AND REFERRALS TO PHYSICIANS AND LAWYERS.

NATIONAL FEDERATION OF PARENTS AND FRIENDS OF LESBIANS AND GAYS (PFLAG)

1101 14TH STREET NW, STE.1030
WASHINGTON, DC 20005
(202) 638-4200
HTTP://WWW.PFLAG.ORG/

INFORMATION AND SUPPORT FOR THOSE WHO CARE ABOUT LESBIAN AND GAY INDIVIDUALS. CONTACTS WITH LOCAL GROUPS PROVIDED. PUBLICATIONS AVAILABLE.

PLANNED PARENTHOOD FEDERATION OF AMERICA

810 SEVENTH AVENUE
NEW YORK, NY 10019
(202) 785-3351 (TO ORDER PUBLICATIONS)
(800) 230-PLAN (230-7526) (FOR CLINIC REFERRALS)

INFORMATION, COUNSELING AND MEDICAL SERVICES RELATED TO REPRODUCTION AND SEXUAL HEALTH PROVIDED WITHOUT REGARD TO ABILITY TO PAY. CHECK PHONE DIRECTORY FOR LOCAL CLINIC LISTINGS.

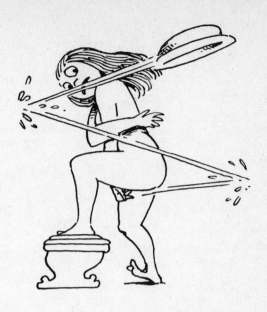

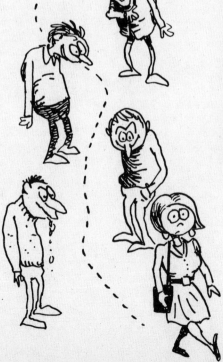

RAPE, ABUSE AND INCEST NATIONAL NETWORK (RAINN)

(800) 656-4673 (656-HOPE)

INFORMATION, COUNSELING AND REFERRALS FOR VICTIMS OF SEXUAL ASSAULT.

SEX INFORMATION AND EDUCATION COUNCIL OF THE UNITED STATES (SIECUS)

130 W. 42ND STREET, STE. 350
NEW YORK, NY 10036
(212) 819-9770
HTTP://WWW.SIECUS.ORG/

AN EDUCATIONAL ORGANIZATION DEDICATED TO PROMOTING HEALTHY SEXUALITY. PROVIDES INFORMATION AND REFERRALS FROM AN EXTENSIVE LIBRARY AND DATABASE. NUMEROUS PUBLICATIONS INCLUDING A MONTHLY JOURNAL.

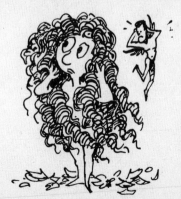

Index

ABOUT THE AUTHORS

CHRISTINE DEVAULT, A FAMILY LIFE EDUCATOR CERTIFIED BY THE NATIONAL COUNCIL ON FAMILY RELATIONS, TEACHES AT CABRILLO COLLEGE IN CALIFORNIA AND HAS WRITTEN WIDELY ON SEXUALITY AND FAMILY LIFE, INCLUDING COAUTHORING TWO TEXTBOOKS. SHE ALSO HAS HAD QUITE A BIT OF FAMILY LIFE EXPERIENCE, HAVING SUCCESSFULLY HERDED THREE CHILDREN THROUGH CHILDHOOD AND ADOLESCENCE. SHE LIVES WITH HER HUSBAND IN SANTA CRUZ, CALIFORNIA, AND TRIES TO SPEND AS MUCH TIME AS POSSIBLE OUTDOORS PHOTOGRAPHING FUZZY ANIMALS.

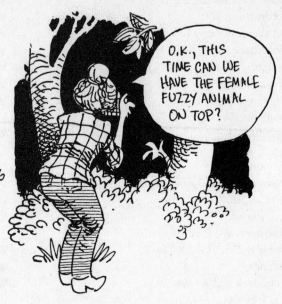

LARRY GONICK, CREATOR OF THE CARTOON GUIDE SERIES, HAS PENNED A GREAT MANY WORKS OF NONFICTION CARTOONING AND IS CURRENTLY STAFF CARTOONIST FOR **MUSE** MAGAZINE. HE LIVES IN SAN FRANCISCO WITH HIS WIFE AND TWO DAUGHTERS. UNTIL RECENTLY, HE DIDN'T QUITE REALIZE THAT AN INTEREST IN SEX COULD BE THOUGHT OF AS AN INTELLECTUAL PURSUIT.

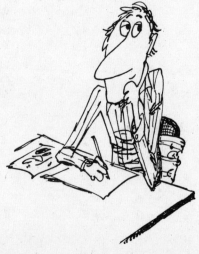